T0263769

Evolving Role of PET-guided Interventional Oncology

Editors

MARNIX G.E.H. LAM
STEPHEN J. HUNT
GHASSAN E. EL-HADDAD
ABASS ALAVI

PET CLINICS

www.pet.theclinics.com

Consulting Editor
ABASS ALAVI

October 2019 • Volume 14 • Number 4

ELSEVIER

1600 John F. Kennedy Boulevard • Suite 1800 • Philadelphia, Pennsylvania, 19103-2899

http://www.pet.theclinics.com

PET CLINICS Volume 14, Number 4
October 2019 ISSN 1556-8598, ISBN-13: 978-0-323-68189-6

Editor: John Vassallo (j.vassallo@elsevier.com)
Developmental Editor: Casey Potter

PET Clinics (ISSN 1556-8598) is published quarterly by Elsevier Inc., 360 Park Avenue South, New York, NY 10010-1710. Months of issue are January, April, July, and October. Periodicals postage paid at New York, NY, and additional mailing offices. Subscription prices per year are $240.00 (US individuals), $396.00 (US institutions), $100.00 (US students), $279.00 (Canadian individuals), $446.00 (Canadian institutions), $140.00 (Canadian students), $275.00 (foreign individuals), $446.00 (foreign institutions), and $140.00 (foreign students). To receive student and resident rate, orders must be accompanied by name of affiliated institution, date of term, and the signature of program/residency coordinator on institution letterhead. Orders will be billed at individual rate until proof of status is received. Foreign air speed delivery is included in all Clinics subscription prices. All prices are subject to change without notice. POSTMASTER: Send address changes to PET Clinics, Elsevier Health Sciences Division, Subscription Customer Service, 3251 Riverport Lane, Maryland Heights, MO 63043. **Customer Service: 1-800-654-2452 (U.S. and Canada); 314-447-8871 (outside U.S. and Canada). Fax: 314-447-8029. E-mail: journalscustomerservice-usa@elsevier.com (for print support); journalsonlinesupport-usa@elsevier.com (for online support).**

Reprints. For copies of 100 or more of articles in this publication, please contact the Commercial Reprints Department, Elsevier Inc., 360 Park Avenue South, New York, NY 10010-1710. Tel.: 212-633-3874; Fax: 212-633-3820; E-mail: reprints@elsevier.com.

PET Clinics is covered in MEDLINE/PubMed (Index Medicus).

Contributors

CONSULTING EDITOR

ABASS ALAVI, MD, MD (Hon), PhD (Hon), DSc (Hon)
Professor of Radiology, Division of Nuclear Medicine, Department of Radiology, Hospital of the University of Pennsylvania, University of Pennsylvania Perelman School of Medicine, Philadelphia, Pennsylvania, USA

EDITORS

MARNIX G.E.H. LAM, MD, PhD
Professor of Nuclear Medicine, Chief of Nuclear Medicine, Department of Radiology and Nuclear Medicine, University Medical Center Utrecht, GA Utrecht, The Netherlands

STEPHEN J. HUNT, MD, PhD, DABR
Assistant Professor of Radiology, Hospital of the University of Pennsylvania, Philadelphia, Pennsylvania, USA

GHASSAN E. EL-HADDAD, MD
Section Head, Radionuclide Therapy Program at H. Lee Moffitt Cancer Center and Research Institute, Associate Member, Diagnostic Imaging and Interventional Radiology Program, Cancer Physiology Program, Associate Professor of Oncologic Sciences at the University of South Florida, Moffitt Cancer Center, Tampa, Florida, USA

ABASS ALAVI, MD, MD (Hon), PhD (Hon), DSc (Hon)
Professor of Radiology, Division of Nuclear Medicine, Department of Radiology, Hospital of the University of Pennsylvania, University of Pennsylvania Perelman School of Medicine, Philadelphia, Pennsylvania, USA

AUTHORS

ABASS ALAVI, MD, MD (Hon), PhD (Hon), DSc (Hon)
Professor of Radiology, Division of Nuclear Medicine, Department of Radiology, Hospital of the University of Pennsylvania, University of Pennsylvania Perelman School of Medicine, Philadelphia, Pennsylvania, USA

CYRUS AYUBCHA, BA
Department of Radiology, Hospital of the University of Pennsylvania, Philadelphia, Pennsylvania, USA

REMCO BASTIAANNET, MSc
Radiology and Nuclear Medicine, University Medical Center Utrecht, Utrecht, Netherlands; The Russell H. Morgan Department of Radiology and Radiological Science, Johns Hopkins School of Medicine, Baltimore, Maryland, USA

TONE FROST BATHEN, PhD
Department of Circulation and Medical Imaging, Norwegian University of Science and Technology, St. Olavs Hospital, Trondheim University Hospital, Trondheim, Norway

HELENA BERTILSSON, MD, PhD
Department of Cancer Research and Molecular Medicine, Norwegian University of Science and Technology, Department of Urology, St. Olavs Hospital, Trondheim University Hospital, Trondheim, Norway

JULIUS CHAPIRO, MD
Department of Radiology and Biomedical Imaging, Yale School of Medicine, New Haven, Connecticut, USA

SIRONG CHEN, PhD
Department of Nuclear Medicine and PET, Medical Physics and Research Department, Hong Kong Sanatorium & Hospital, Happy Valley, Hong Kong, China

SHING KEE CHEUNG, MBBS
Department of Nuclear Medicine and PET, Hong Kong Sanatorium & Hospital, Happy Valley, Hong Kong, China

HUGO W.A.M. DE JONG, PhD
Radiology and Nuclear Medicine, University Medical Center Utrecht, Utrecht, Netherlands

MICHAEL J. DRABKIN, MD
Interventional Radiology Service, Memorial Sloan Kettering Cancer, New York, New York, USA

MATTIJS ELSCHOT, PhD
Department of Circulation and Medical Imaging, Norwegian University of Science and Technology, Department of Radiology and Nuclear Medicine, St. Olavs Hospital, Trondheim University Hospital, Trondheim, Norway

CHI LAI HO, MD
Department of Nuclear Medicine and PET, Hong Kong Sanatorium & Hospital, Happy Valley, Hong Kong, China

STEPHEN J. HUNT, MD, PhD, DABR
Assistant Professor of Radiology, Hospital of the University of Pennsylvania, Philadelphia, Pennsylvania, USA

HÅKON JOHANSEN, MD
Department of Radiology and Nuclear Medicine, St. Olavs Hospital, Trondheim University Hospital, Trondheim, Norway

SIRISH A. KISHORE, MD
Assistant Professor of Radiology, Weill-Cornell Medical College, Assistant Member, Department of Radiology, Division of Interventional Radiology, Memorial Sloan Kettering Cancer Center, New York, New York, USA

MARNIX G.E.H. LAM, MD, PhD
Professor of Nuclear Medicine, Chief of Nuclear Medicine, Department of Radiology and Nuclear Medicine, University Medical Center Utrecht, GA Utrecht, The Netherlands

SVERRE LANGØRGEN, MD
Department of Radiology and Nuclear Medicine, St. Olavs Hospital, Trondheim University Hospital, Trondheim, Norway

THOMAS WAI TONG LEUNG, MD
Comprehensive Oncology Center, Hong Kong Sanatorium & Hospital, Happy Valley, Hong Kong, China

MARTIN A. LODGE, MS, PhD
Radiology and Nuclear Medicine, University Medical Center Utrecht, Utrecht, Netherlands; The Russell H. Morgan Department of Radiology and Radiological Science, Johns Hopkins School of Medicine, Baltimore, Maryland, USA

HESSE MICHEL, PhD
Nuclear Medicine, Cliniques Universitaires Saint-Luc, Brussels, Belgium

DARKO PUCAR, MD, PhD
Department of Radiology and Biomedical Imaging, Yale School of Medicine, New Haven, Connecticut, USA

LAWRENCE SAPERSTEIN, MD
Department of Radiology and Biomedical Imaging, Yale School of Medicine, New Haven, Connecticut, USA

LYNN JEANETTE SAVIC, MD
Department of Radiology and Biomedical Imaging, Yale School of Medicine, New Haven, Connecticut, USA; Institute of Radiology, Charité - Universitätsmedizin Berlin, Corporate Member of Freie Universität Berlin, Humboldt-Universität, Berlin Institute of Health, Berlin, Germany

ISABEL SCHOBERT, BS
Department of Radiology and Biomedical
Imaging, Yale School of Medicine,
New Haven, Connecticut, USA; Institute
of Radiology, Charité - Universitätsmedizin
Berlin, Corporate Member of Freie
Universität Berlin, Humboldt-Universität,
Berlin Institute of Health, Berlin,
Germany

KIRSTEN MARGRETE SELNÆS, PhD
Department of Radiology and
Nuclear Medicine, St. Olavs Hospital,
Trondheim University Hospital, Trondheim,
Norway

SIAVASH MEHDIZADEH SERAJ, MD
Department of Radiology, Hospital
of the University of Pennsylvania,
Philadelphia, Pennsylvania,
USA

**CONSTANTINOS T. SOFOCLEOUS, MD,
PhD, FSIR, FCIRSE**
Professor of Interventional Radiology,
Weill-Cornell Medical College, Attending
Physician, Interventional Oncology, Memorial
Sloan Kettering Cancer Center, New York,
New York, USA

WALRAND STEPHAN, PhD
Nuclear Medicine, Cliniques Universitaires
Saint-Luc, Brussels, Belgium

TORGRIM TANDSTAD, MD, PhD
Department of Cancer Research and Molecular
Medicine, Norwegian University of Science and
Technology, The Cancer Clinic, St. Olavs
Hospital, Trondheim University Hospital,
Trondheim, Norway

MAHDI ZIRAKCHIAN ZADEH, MD, MHM
Department of Radiology, Hospital of the
University of Pennsylvania, Children's Hospital
of Philadelphia, Philadelphia, Pennsylvania,
USA

Contents

Interventional radiology procedures have revolutionized the treatment of cancer and interventional oncology is now the fourth pillar of cancer care. The article discusses the importance of fluorodeoxyglucose (FDG)-PET imaging, and dual time-point imaging in the context of PET/computed tomography as applied to treatments of liver malignancy. The necessary paradigm shift in the adoption of novel segmentation methodologies to express global disease burden is explored.

PET has become an essential tool for staging and response assessment in oncologic imaging. Over the past decade it has also evolved into a tool for image-guided interventions, specifically in the rapidly growing field of interventional oncology. PET-guided biopsies have greater sensitivity and diagnostic yield for fluorodeoxyglucose-avid lesions. Real-time PET imaging can also provide valuable image guidance during therapeutic minimally invasive procedures such as ablation of PET-avid tumors. The increasing use of PET in the assessment of therapeutic response results in earlier identification of disease that is amenable to image-guided therapies.

Response to transarterial chemoembolization (TACE) in patients with liver cancer is commonly assessed on MRI or CT to quantify tumor necrosis and morphologic changes that occur gradually. However, the efficacy of embolotherapies remains limited because of local recurrence, as treated tumors demonstrate individual molecular characteristics that alter susceptibility and response to embolotherapies. Upregulation of cancer cell glycolysis can be detected by fluorine-18-fluorodeoxyglucose PET. Therefore, the combination of functional (PET) with commonly used cross-sectional imaging techniques (MRI, CT) can help characterize and monitor liver tumors with the potential to improve TACE toward becoming a more personalized and tumor microenvironment-directed therapy.

Recent research into the efficacy of radioembolization has brought this field to an interesting position, in which fluorodeoxyglucose (FDG)-PET/CT is being used extensively for prognosis and response assessment, as well as a tool to define viable tumor volumes for the use in dosimetry. As such, there is an overlap with existing techniques used in radiotherapy; however, many are very specific to the radioembolization paradigm. This article describes the current state-of-the-art of the use of FDG-PET/CT for patient selection, prognosis, treatment evaluation, and as a research tool into absorbed dose-response relationships in radioembolization.

Pretreatment dual-tracer (^{18}F-fluorodeoxyglucose and ^{11}C-acetate) PET/computed tomography (CT) has potential to predict treatment response for ^{90}Y microsphere radioembolization (RE) in patients with inoperable hepatocellular carcinoma (HCC). Patients with ^{11}C-acetate-avid HCC have a better response to ^{90}Y microsphere RE, and possibly better survival. Pretreatment dual-tracer PET/CT has a significant theranostic value on ^{90}Y microsphere RE in determining target tumor dose for HCCs with different cellular differentiation, metabolic tumor volume, and functioning liver volume, and can be used to prescribe individual injected activity of ^{90}Y microspheres.

This article presents a comprehensive review of the ^{90}Y PET/CT challenges in imaging post liver radioembolization. Specificities of the different PET systems are identified. Conclusions are drawn to help the design of phantom validation studies, quantification of intrahepatic activity, assessment of tumor dosimetry, and checking of extrahepatic sphere delivery in clinical routine.

Interventional oncology treatments have profound effects on tumor immunity. Quantitative molecular imaging with FDG-PET has the potential to aid in understanding baseline tumor characteristics that can predict response to interventional oncology treatments and immunotherapy. This review highlights some of the evidence for immune activation in the setting of locoregional therapies, and the patterns of treatment response that may be expected in the setting of immune induction. Also presented is an argument for measuring global disease metabolic activity over conventional methods of PET quantitation to circumvent challenges in correlating conventional methods of PET quantification to overall disease activity.

This article presents an overview of the current literature on PET imaging with prostate-specific membrane antigen ligands, especially focusing on the potential role of simultaneous PET/magnetic resonance imaging for the planning of salvage radiotherapy in patients with prostate cancer with biochemical recurrence after radical prostatectomy.

PET CLINICS

THE CLINICS ARE AVAILABLE ONLINE!
Access your subscription at:
www.theclinics.com

PROGRAM OBJECTIVE

The goal of the *PET Clinics* is to keep practicing radiologists and radiology residents up to date with current clinical practice in positron emission tomography by providing timely articles reviewing the state of the art in patient care.

TARGET AUDIENCE

Practicing radiologists, radiology residents, and other health care professionals who provide patient care utilizing radiologic findings.

LEARNING OBJECTIVES

Upon completion of this activity, participants will be able to:

1. Review challenges inherent to ^{90}Y PET/CT imaging in radioembolization.
2. Discuss the current and evolving roles of PET in interventional oncology.
3. Recognize the current role and possible future applications of PET in the diagnosis of primary and secondary liver malignancies and monitoring of tumor response to TACE.

ACCREDITATION

The Elsevier Office of Continuing Medical Education (EOCME) is accredited by the Accreditation Council for Continuing Medical Education (ACCME) to provide continuing medical education for physicians.

The EOCME designates this journal-based CME activity for a maximum of 8 *AMA PRA Category 1 Credit*(s)™. Physicians should claim only the credit commensurate with the extent of their participation in the activity.

All other health care professionals requesting continuing education credit for this enduring material will be issued a certificate of participation.

DISCLOSURE OF CONFLICTS OF INTEREST

The EOCME assesses conflict of interest with its instructors, faculty, planners, and other individuals who are in a position to control the content of CME activities. All relevant conflicts of interest that are identified are thoroughly vetted by EOCME for fair balance, scientific objectivity, and patient care recommendations. EOCME is committed to providing its learners with CME activities that promote improvements or quality in healthcare and not a specific proprietary business or a commercial interest.

The planning committee, staff, authors and editors listed below have identified no financial relationships or relationships to products or devices they or their spouse/life partner have with commercial interest related to the content of this CME activity:

Abass Alavi, MD, MD (Hon), PhD (Hon), DSc (Hon); Cyrus Ayubcha, BA; Remco Bastiaannet, MSc; Tone Frost Bathen, PhD; Helena Bertilsson, MD, PhD; Julius Chapiro, MD; Sirong Chen, PhD; Shing Kee Cheung, MBBS; Hugo W.A.M. de Jong, PhD; Michael J. Drabkin, MD; Ghassan El-Haddad, MD; Mattijs Elschot, PhD; Hesse Michel, PhD; Chi Lai Ho, MD; Stephen J. Hunt, MD, PhD, DABR; Håkon Johansen, MD; Alison Kemp; Sirish A. Kishore, MD; Thomas Wai Tong Leung, MD; Martin A. Lodge, MSc, PhD; Darko Pucar, MD, PhD; Lawrence Saperstein, MD; Lynn Jeanette Savic, MD; Isabel Schobert, BS; Kirsten Margrete Selnæs, PhD; Siavash Mehdizadeh Seraj, MD; Torgrim Tandstad, MD, PhD; John Vassallo; Vignesh Viswanathan; Walrand Stephan, PhD; Mahdi Zirakchian Zadeh, MD, MHM.

The planning committee, staff, authors and editors listed below have identified financial relationships or relationships to products or devices they or their spouse/life partner have with commercial interest related to the content of this CME activity:

Marnix G.E.H. Lam, MD, PhD: receives research support from Quirem Medical BV; is a consultant/advisor and receives research support from BTG International Ltd and Terumo Medical Corporation

Constantinos T. Sofocleous, MD, PhD, FSIR, FCIRSE: receives research support from BTG International Ltd; is a consultant/advisor for General Electric Company and Terumo Medical Corporation; receives research support and is a consultant/advisor for Medical Devices Business Services, Inc.

UNAPPROVED/OFF-LABEL USE DISCLOSURE

The EOCME requires CME faculty to disclose to the participants:

1. When products or procedures being discussed are off-label, unlabelled, experimental, and/or investigational (not US Food and Drug Administration [FDA] approved); and
2. Any limitations on the information presented, such as data that are preliminary or that represent ongoing research, interim analyses, and/or unsupported opinions. Faculty may discuss information about pharmaceutical agents that is outside of FDA-approved labelling. This information is intended solely for CME and is not intended to promote off-label use of these medications. If you have any questions, contact the medical affairs department of the manufacturer for the most recent prescribing information.

TO ENROLL

To enroll in the *PET Clinics* Continuing Medical Education program, call customer service at 1-800-654-2452 or sign up online at http://www.theclinics.com/home/cme. The CME program is available to subscribers for an additional annual fee of USD $235.

METHOD OF PARTICIPATION

In order to claim credit, participants must complete the following:

1. Complete enrolment as indicated above.
2. Read the activity.
3. Complete the CME Test and Evaluation. Participants must achieve a score of 70% on the test. All CME Tests and Evaluations must be completed online.

CME INQUIRIES/SPECIAL NEEDS

For all CME inquiries or special needs, please contact elsevierCME@elsevier.com.

Preface

Evolving Role of PET in Interventional Radiology-Based Oncology Procedures

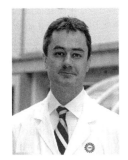

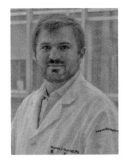

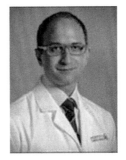

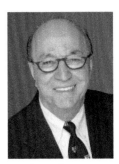

Marnix G.E.H. Lam, MD, PhD   Stephen J. Hunt, MD, PhD   Ghassan E. El-Haddad, MD   Abass Alavi, MD

Editors

Interventional oncology has become an integral fourth pillar in the treatment of cancer over the past few decades. Interventional oncology is a set of locoregional oncologic therapies delivered by interventional radiologists for the treatment of solid tumor deposits. Traditional morphologic imaging methods of staging disease and measuring treatment response are not designed to measure locoregional tumor responses or global treatment responses in the setting of locoregional therapy. For example, if a patient has liver-dominant metastatic disease, which represents the primary site of tumor progression, locoregional therapy may provide a clinical benefit that cannot be predicted or assessed by conventional morphologic methods of tumor response or progression. As medical oncology expands treatment options away from conventional broadly cytotoxic chemotherapies toward more targeted therapies, tumor clonal escape mechanisms result in locoregional progression that does not represent a "global" treatment failure, but rather limited "isolated" sites of progression. This limited progression, so-called oligometastatic disease, has been demonstrated to respond well to locoregional therapies, including percutaneous ablation, transarterial chemoembolization (TACE), transarterial radioembolization (TARE),

and high-dose ablative radiotherapy. Conventional imaging methodologies are not designed to predict and measure treatment response.

In this issue, we hope to illustrate the role of PET in informing locoregional treatment choice, including predicting response to treatment, intraprocedural PET treatment use, and its use in measuring treatment response. While there still exist inherent limitations to using conventional PET parameters for these indications, Seraj and colleagues provide evidence that the accuracy of PET quantification can be enhanced by adopting novel quantitative techniques that can better reflect global disease burden. Sofocleus and colleagues provide an overview of the use of PET with fludeoxyglucose (FDG-PET) in ablation, including its expanding use intraprocedurally to provide a real-time measure of complete tumor treatment. Savic and colleagues review the potential for FDG-PET to improve TACE to be a more personalized and tumor microenvironment–directed therapy. Dr Lam and colleagues describe the current state-of-the-art use of FDG-PET/computed tomography (CT) for patient selection, prognosis, and treatment evaluation in the setting of Y90 radioembolization (TARE). Dr Leung and colleagues provide evidence that pretreatment

PET Clin 14 (2019) xiii–xiv
https://doi.org/10.1016/j.cpet.2019.07.001
1556-8598/19/© 2019 Published by Elsevier Inc.

dual-tracer (^{18}F-FDG and ^{11}C-acetate) PET/CT has the potential to predict treatment response for TARE in patients with inoperable hepatocellular carcinoma (HCC), and in particular, has a significant theranostic value in determining target tumor dose for HCC. Dr Walrand and colleagues provide a comprehensive review of the specific challenges inherent to direct PET imaging of Y90 microspheres, including its intrahepatic and extrahepatic quantitation and technical factors that can limit its accuracy. Immunotherapy has been the most recent advance in targeted therapies, which has demonstrated significant improvements in treatment response and has generated nearly unbridled enthusiasm in the oncology community. Unfortunately, conventional imaging measures of treatment response and immunologic response are inadequate and often inaccurate for measuring response in the setting of immunotherapy. Dr Hunt and colleagues provide evidence that FDG-PET has the potential to aid in both predicting and measuring immunologic treatment response in the setting of locoregional therapies. Prostate cancer treatment in recent years has expanded beyond prostatectomy and hormone ablation to more use of locoregional treatment modalities, including magnetic resonance (MR)-guided ablation, high-intensity focused ultrasound, and high-dose radiotherapy. In the final article of this issue, Dr Bathen and colleagues present an overview of the current literature on PET imaging with prostate-specific membrane antigen ligands, especially focusing on the potential role of simultaneous PET/MR imaging for the planning of salvage radiotherapy in patients with biochemical recurrence after radical prostatectomy. In summary, we hope you find this issue informative, and that the articles herein pique the interest of the oncology clinical and research community to expand the research and clinical use of PET imaging in cancer care.

Marnix G.E.H. Lam, MD, PhD
Department of Radiology and Nuclear Medicine
University Medical Center Utrecht
Kamernummer E.01.1.29
Huispostnummer E01.132
Postbus 85500
3508 GA Utrecht, The Netherlands

Stephen J. Hunt, MD, PhD
Hospital of the University of Pennsylvania
Ground Dulles
3400 Spruce Street
Philadelphia, PA 19104, USA

Ghassan E. El-Haddad, MD
Radionuclide Therapy Program at
H. Lee Moffitt Cancer Center and
Research Institute
Diagnostic Imaging &
Interventional Radiology Program
Cancer Physiology Program
University of South Florida
Moffitt Cancer Center
12902 USF Magnolia Drive
Tampa, FL 33612, USA

Abass Alavi, MD
Department of Radiology
Hospital of the University of Pennsylvania
3400 Spruce Street
Philadelphia, PA 19104, USA

E-mail addresses:
M.Lam@umcutrecht.nl (M.G.E.H. Lam)
stephen.hunt@uphs.upenn.edu (S.J. Hunt)
gassnucmed@gmail.com (G.E. El-Haddad)
Abass.Alavi@uphs.upenn.edu (A. Alavi)

The Evolving Role of PET-Based Novel Quantitative Techniques in the Interventional Radiology Procedures of the Liver

Siavash Mehdizadeh Seraj, MD[a], Cyrus Ayubcha, BA[a],
Mahdi Zirakchian Zadeh, MD, MHM[a,b],
Abass Alavi, MD, MD(Hon), PhD(Hon), DSc(Hon)[a,*], Stephen J. Hunt, MD, PhD, DABR[a]

KEYWORDS

- FDG-PET ● Quantification ● Dual time-point imaging ● Interventional radiology ● Liver ● Malignancy

KEY POINTS

- Fluorodeoxyglucose (FDG)-PET/computed tomography has an expanding role in the interventional radiology procedures of the liver.
- The quantitative analyses of FDG-PET have shown the ability to assess treatment response and prognosis.
- The accuracy of PET quantification can be enhanced by adopting novel quantitative techniques that can better reflect global disease burden.

INTRODUCTION

Interventional radiology (IR) procedures have revolutionized the treatment of cancer and given birth to the emerging field of interventional oncology (IO) as the fourth pillar of cancer care. These procedures have been used both as palliative and curative treatments in a variety of malignancies.[1–4] Several established IO treatment options, such as radiofrequency ablation (RFA), transarterial chemoembolization (TACE), transarterial radioembolization (TARE), and high-intensity focused ultrasonography, have demonstrated efficacy in treating hepatic tumors. These noninvasive procedures often improve the clinical outcome of patients with primary hepatic tumors, as well as metastatic hepatic tumors.[2] However, an individualized assessment is required to determine the optimal treatment plan for a patient. Moreover, accurate tools are needed to monitor the response to treatment to evaluate the efficacy of the treatment and patient's subsequent management planning.

Fluorodeoxyglucose (FDG)-PET imaging was first conceived in the early 1970s by researchers at the University of Pennsylvania as a means of noninvasively measuring brain's function and metabolism.[5] Initially, FDG-PET was predominantly used for the early detection and assessment of various neurologic disorders.[6,7] Soon thereafter, the application of this imaging modality was expanded as FDG-PET became a prominent technique for diagnosis, staging, treatment response monitoring, and prognosis of different malignancies.[8] An advantage of FDG-PET is the ability to quantify the magnitude of radiotracer uptake, which is representative of disease burden. A

[a] Department of Radiology, Hospital of University of Pennsylvania, 3400 Spruce street, Philadelphia, PA 19104, USA; [b] Department of Radiology, Children's Hospital of Philadelphia, 3401 Civic Center Boulevard, Philadelphia, PA 19104, USA
* Corresponding author. 3400 Spruce Street, Philadelphia, PA 19104.
E-mail address: abass.alavi@uphs.upenn.edu

PET Clin 14 (2019) 419–425
https://doi.org/10.1016/j.cpet.2019.06.004
1556-8598/19/© 2019 Elsevier Inc. All rights reserved.

common parameter of tracer uptake is maximum standardized uptake value (SUV$_{max}$), which is corrected for the injection dose and the patient's weight. However, the reliability of SUV$_{max}$ has been questioned and mean standardized uptake value (SUV$_{mean}$) has been suggested to be a superior measure of tracer uptake because it is not the value of a single voxel but rather the average of all voxels within a lesion.[9] There are other considerations that may improve the utility of FDG-PET quantification, such as dual time-point imaging (DTPI), incorporating the tumor's volumetric data; partial volume correction; and, most importantly, the global disease assessment approach. In this article, the importance of these advanced quantification techniques is discussed in the context of PET/computed tomography (CT) as applied to IO treatments of liver malignancy. Furthermore, the necessity for a paradigm shift in the adoption of novel segmentation methodologies to express global disease burden is explored.

ROLE OF QUALITATIVE PET/COMPUTED TOMOGRAPHY IN INTERVENTIONAL RADIOLOGY PROCEDURES OF THE LIVER

Quantitative and qualitative analyses of FDG-PET/CT have an expanding role in the IO treatment of the liver malignancies. The initial utility of FDG-PET/CT in such procedures is determining which patients will benefit from said therapeutic techniques.[10] The reason for this is the superiority of FDG-PET/CT compared with structural modalities in detecting early extrahepatic metastasis that leads to a change in tumor staging and, subsequently, a change in treatment plan.[10] Using a sequential algorithm, Denecke and colleagues[11] explored the comparative utility of different radiological modalities and techniques in the process of subject selection for yttrium-90 (Y-90) TARE. They found that CT alone was insufficient in excluding extrahepatic disease, and FDG-PET along with MR imaging was more sensitive in identifying extrahepatic lesions absent on CT.[11] In

another investigation, CT and FDG PET/CT modalities were compared with assessing the added diagnostic value of FDG-PET/CT during subjects' treatment planning before Y-90 TARE.[12] The treatment strategies of 7 out of 42 (17%) subjects were changed with the addition of FDG-PET due to the detection of extrahepatic metastasis in 6 subjects and an intrahepatic lesion in 1 subject (**Fig. 1**).

ROLE OF QUANTITATIVE PET/COMPUTED TOMOGRAPHY IN INTERVENTIONAL RADIOLOGY PROCEDURES OF THE LIVER

The presence of distant metastases can be visually confirmed by FDG-PET. The quantitative techniques of FDG-PET can provide additional benefit during prognosis evaluation and treatment response monitoring. Various studies have demonstrated the prognostic value of FDG-PET parameters in subjects undergoing IR procedures.[13–18] In a prospective study of hepatocellular carcinoma (HCC) subjects undergoing Y-90 transarterial embolization, lesion-derived SUV$_{max}$ and tumor-to-liver uptake ratio (lesion's SUV$_{max}$ divided by the healthy liver's SUV$_{mean}$) were found to be prognostic factors with respect to survival in these subjects.[16] Piduru and colleagues[15] evaluated the prognostic value of pretreatment FDG-PET/CT scans in subjects with hepatic melanoma metastasis undergoing Y-90 TARE. They concluded that metabolic tumor burden, as derived by the division of metabolic tumor volume (MTV) by total liver volume, was associated with inferior survival.[15] SUV$_{max}$ failed to significantly predict the survival of these subjects.[15] A recent study explored the ability of 11c-acetate and FDG PET/CT to predict the treatment response and prognosis after TACE in HCC subjects.[14] Subsequent univariate analysis indicated that tumor uptake normalized by liver uptake (TNR)-FDG (tumor SUV$_{max}$ to healthy liver SUV$_{mean}$) significantly predicted treatment response after TACE.[14] Both univariate and multivariate analyses found that TNR-FDG predicted recurrence after TACE.[14]

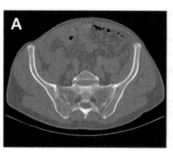 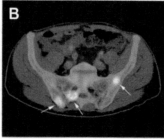

Fig. 1. Multiple bone metastases. (*A*) The abdominal CT (bone window) with no evidence of involvement of the bone. (*B*) An FDG-PET image with multiple focal hotspots in the pelvis (*arrows*). This patient was excluded from treatment because of multiple bone metastases seen on FDG-PET that had not been detected on abdominal CT. (*From* Rosenbaum CE, van den Bosch MA, Veldhuis WB, et al. Added value of FDG-PET imaging in the diagnostic workup for yttrium-90 radioembolisation in patients with colorectal cancer liver metastases. European radiology. 2013;23(4):931-7.)

Accurate assessment of the response to tumor ablation or embolization is vital. Studies have shown that FDG-PET is more sensitive than CT or MR imaging in identifying local recurrence after RFA or cryoablation in liver metastatic lesions.[19–21] It has also been shown that the percentage change of the tumor's SUV_{max} between baseline and early interim FDG-PET/CT is predictive of overall survival and time to progression in HCC subjects treated with TACE.[21] The results indicate that FDG-PET/CT might be a valuable imaging technique for treatment response assessment and prognosis for HCC patients treated with TACE.[21] Responders to Y-90 TARE characterized by decrease in peak standardized uptake value (SUV_{peak}) and total lesion glycolysis (TLG) according to Positron Emission Tomography Response Criteria in Solid Tumors (PERCIST) have been demonstrated to have longer overall survival, progression-free survival, and time to intrahepatic progression.[22] More recently, evidence suggests that new quantitative parameters, including volumetric tumor data, may be more accurate and sensitive in prognosis evaluation of patients treating with Y-90 radioembolization.[13,23,24]

THE NECESSITY OF USING A NOVEL QUANTITATIVE APPROACH IN INTERVENTIONAL RADIOLOGY PROCEDURES

Currently, the quantitative assessment of PET images mostly relies on assigning regions of interest (ROI) to a lesser area of the overall lesion to derive relevant uptake measures of the disease activity. The most common parameter used in this conventional method is SUV_{max}. Unfortunately, this conventional approach suffers from a variety of shortcomings that may engender misleading results. Sampling a portion of an active disease fails to accurately reflect whole disease burden.

Moreover, the use of SUV_{max}-derived parameters further introduces variability because most malignant tumors are heterogeneous and SUV_{max} represents a single voxel of activity in the greater region of overall tumor burden. Furthermore, SUV_{max} is likely to deviate due to noise and motion,[25] and the SUV_{max} can be altered by contamination from the adjacent tissues. In addition, ROI assignment on just a portion of the disease is an operator-dependent procedure because there are no consistent protocols regarding the manner of ROI placement; such inherent interreader variation results in fundamentally nonreproducible values. Another issue with conventional methods of PET quantification involves the absence of partial volume correction, which is important because of the limited spatial resolution of PET scanners. Studies have previously demonstrated that partial volume correction can provide more accurate measures of lesion metabolic status.[26] The partial volume effect is a serious factor, especially for smaller malignant lesions, which disperses the true magnitude of uptake into a larger area so that the measured uptake (ie, SUV) will be invariably lower than the true uptake of the lesion.[27] This will lead to measurement errors and, when 2 scans are required,[27] such as treatment response monitoring with FDG-PET for IR procedures, the impact will be doubled. Therefore, adopting a new approach that accounts for the partial volume correction during the quantitative analysis of FDG-PET is paramount.

Novel advanced software and developed methods of PET segmentation and quantification have been asserted to address these shortcomings. Semiautomated methods of quantification have been introduced to better estimate the PET parameters such as SUV_{mean}, SUV_{max}, MTV, TLG, and partial volume corrected TLG (pvcTLG), which are useful in accurately determining disease burden or treatment response[9,28] **Figs. 2** and **3** These

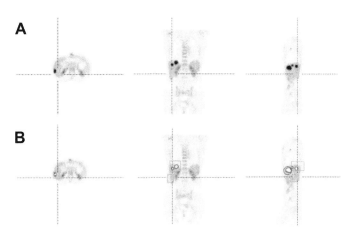

A

B

Fig. 2. FDG-PET images of a 66-year-old woman with metastatic liver disease before Y-90 radioembolization treatment. (*A*) Pretreatment FDG-PET images in the axial, coronal, and sagittal planes demonstrate abnormal increased FDG uptake in the liver. (*B*) The same PET images after segmentation of all active lesions using the adaptive thresholding system of ROVER software (ABX, Radeberg, Germany).

A   **B**

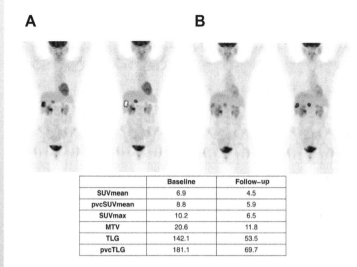

	Baseline	Follow-up
SUVmean	6.9	4.5
pvcSUVmean	8.8	5.9
SUVmax	10.2	6.5
MTV	20.6	11.8
TLG	142.1	53.5
pvcTLG	181.1	69.7

Fig. 3. Illustration of a method to quantify the global disease burden and treatment response in a 38-year-old woman with invasive ductal carcinoma metastases to the liver. (*A*) Pretreatment FDG-PET scan 60 minutes following the FDG administration. (*B*) FDG-PET scan of the same patient after TACE treatment. The scans were analyzed using the ROVER software. PET parameters, including SUV_{mean}, partial volume corrected ($pvcSUV_{mean}$), SUV_{max}, MTV, TLG, and pvcTLG were obtained and changes between baseline and follow-up are noted.

parameters derived from the semiautomatic algorithm of the software incorporate all avid lesions to better express the global disease burden.[9] An advantage of including all available lesions, in other words, a global disease assessment, is the ability to express true disease burden throughout the body. Furthermore, the semiautomatic nature of this method reduces the operator-dependency inherent in other techniques and, accordingly, more reproducible results can be obtained. This reproducibility is vital when using SUV_{mean}-based parameters because SUV_{mean} is sensitive to the particular area or volume of the relevant ROI.[25] The consistent and reproducible application of ROIs on all lesions by this semiautomated technique increases the reproducibility of SUV_{mean}. The other advantage of this approach is that it allows for obtaining the volumetric parameters of PET quantification, namely MTV, TLG, and pvcTLG. These novel PET-based quantitative parameters have shown promise in the prognostic evaluation of many oncologic scenarios.[26,29–31] Recently, Seraj and colleagues[13] have shown that the volumetric PET parameters derived from the incorporation of all active lesions were predictive of progression-free survival and overall survival in subjects undergoing Y-90 TARE. Results of this study indicate the feasibility of applying the global disease assessment in the evaluation of patients undergoing IR procedures of the liver. Therefore, it may be appropriate to use this global quantitative approach to the PET scans of patients receiving IO based therapies.

DUAL TIME-POINT IMAGING

DTPI was first introduced in 2001 by Zhuang and colleagues[32] in an attempt to differentiate malignant lesions from benign lesions. DTPI uses the principle that inflammatory and infectious lesions' FDG uptake declines over time, whereas, in malignant lesions, FDG accumulation consistently increases for several hours following the tracer injection.[33–37] Additionally, the delayed imaging can detect malignant lesions that may not have appeared sufficiently avid on early time-point scans.[38,39] Delayed imaging is most useful in organs that eliminate FDG more rapidly, such as liver.[40] As many studies have shown, the amount of FDG activity in the normal liver decreases over time[40–44] and malignant lesions tend to retain FDG, thus, the increased contrast between normal hepatic tissue and the malignant tumor over time bolsters the detection of malignancies in the liver. Such enhanced detection has been confirmed by 2 separate prospective studies that assessed the utility of delayed imaging in detecting hepatic metastasis.[39,45] In the first study, 53 out of 90 proven cases of metastatic lesions in the liver were detected correctly on standard imaging. However, delayed images were able to detect 81 of the 90 metastatic lesions, meaning that 30% of the verified lesions were detectable only on delayed imaging[45] (**Figs. 4** and **5**). In the second study, 79 malignant hepatic lesions were confirmed and standard early time-point images were able to detect 57 of the 79 lesions, whereas 66 of the 79 lesions were detected in the delayed scan.[39] The sensitivity and specificity of standard early time-point imaging in the diagnosis of the hepatic metastasis were 81% and 91%, respectively. The sensitivity and specificity of delayed time-point imaging in the diagnosis of the hepatic metastases were 91% and 95%, respectively.[39] At this delayed time-point, not only can intrahepatic malignant lesions be better visualized but the extrahepatic malignant lesions are also more likely

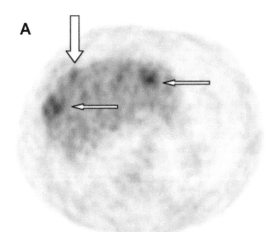

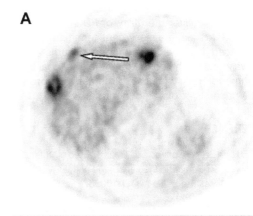

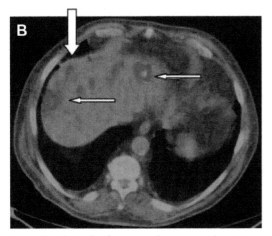

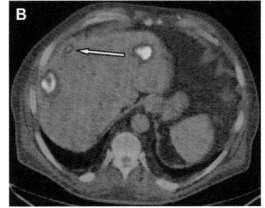

Fig. 5. (*A, B*) On the second delayed scan, a third metastasis could be detected (*arrow*) with an increased SUV and a higher tumor-to-background ratio compared with the first scan. (*From* Dirisamer A, Halpern BS, Schima W, Heinisch M, Wolf F, Beheshti M, et al. Dual-time-point FDG-PET/CT for the detection of hepatic metastases. Molecular Imaging and Biology. 2008;10(6):335-40.)

Fig. 4. (*A, B*) On the first scan, there are at least 2 metastases (*small arrows*) and some inhomogeneous lesions (*large arrow*) with a low SUV that cannot be differentiated from normal liver tissue uptake. (*From* Dirisamer A, Halpern BS, Schima W, Heinisch M, Wolf F, Beheshti M, et al. Dual-time-point FDG-PET/CT for the detection of hepatic metastases. Molecular Imaging and Biology. 2008;10(6):335-40; with permission.)

to be detected.[46] These observations imply that DTPI offers radiologists the ideal medium to identify intrahepatic lesions or extrahepatic metastasis and better optimize IR treatment plan selection.

Researchers have further investigated the role of DTPI in treatment response assessment.[47] Taghvaei and colleagues[47] studied the correlation between ΔSUV_{mean} ([delayed SUV_{mean} of lesion - early SUV_{mean} of lesion] early SUV_{mean} of lesion) in multiple myeloma lesions before treatment with tumor treatment response to chemotherapy. The study determined that in pretreatment DTPI scans elevated ΔSUV_{mean} was found in those lesions with partial response, whereas lower ΔSUV_{mean} was found in lesions with complete response to treatment.[47] This implies that DTPI

can enhance the accuracy of prognosis because increasing FDG retention may indicate more aggressive forms of malignancy. Similar studies in the context of IO treatment are necessary to further elaborate the role of DTPI per respective IO procedure.

SUMMARY

As the role of FDG-PET/CT continues to grow in IO, the shortcomings of present measurement techniques must be addressed to optimize the utility of this imaging modality. FDG-PET/CT has been shown to be superior in detection of extrahepatic metastasis compared with structural imaging studies such as CT. The quantitative assessment of PET has a potentially significant role in the prognosis and treatment response evaluation in IO procedures. Other techniques, such as partial volume correction, DTPI, and global disease assessment may further bolster the utility of FDG-PET. Given that global disease assessment techniques have been used in several analogous circumstances and validated in the context of other malignancies, it is time to apply this novel quantitative approach to IO-based liver-directed therapies.

REFERENCES

1. O'Neill SB, O'Connor OJ, Ryan MF, et al. Interventional radiology and the care of the oncology patient. Radiol Res Pract 2011;2011:160867.

2. Loffroy R, Estivalet L, Favelier S, et al. Interventional radiology therapies for liver cancer. Hepatoma Res 2016;2:1–9.

3. Lee W-K, Lau EW, Chin K, et al. Modern diagnostic and therapeutic interventional radiology in lung cancer. J Thorac Dis 2013;5(Suppl 5):S511.

4. Campbell TC, Roenn JH. Palliative Care for Interventional Radiology: An Oncologist's Perspective. Semin Intervent Radiol 2007;24(4):375–81.

5. Alavi A, Reivich M. Guest editorial: the conception of FDG-PET imaging. Semin Nucl Med 2002;32(1):2–5.

6. Alavi A, Dann R, Chawluk J, et al. Positron emission tomography imaging of regional cerebral glucose metabolism. Semin Nucl Med 1986;16(1):2–34.

7. Alavi A, Reivich M, Greenberg J, et al. Mapping of functional activity in brain with 18F-fluoro-deoxyglucose. Semin Nucl Med 1981;11(1):24–31.

8. Hess S, Blomberg BA, Zhu HJ, et al. The pivotal role of FDG-PET/CT in modern medicine. Acad Radiol 2014;21(2):232–49.

9. Basu S, Zaidi H, Salavati A, et al. FDG PET/CT methodology for evaluation of treatment response in lymphoma: from "graded visual analysis" and "semi-quantitative SUVmax" to global disease burden assessment. Eur J Nucl Med Mol Imaging 2014;41(11):2158–60.

10. Samim M, El-Haddad GE, Molenaar IQ, et al. [18F] Fluorodeoxyglucose PET for interventional oncology in liver malignancy. PET Clin 2014;9(4):469–95.

11. Denecke T, Rühl R, Hildebrandt B, et al. Planning transarterial radioembolization of colorectal liver metastases with Yttrium 90 microspheres: evaluation of a sequential diagnostic approach using radiologic and nuclear medicine imaging techniques. Eur Radiol 2008;18(5):892–902.

12. Rosenbaum CE, van den Bosch MA, Veldhuis WB, et al. Added value of FDG-PET imaging in the diagnostic workup for yttrium-90 radioembolisation in patients with colorectal cancer liver metastases. Eur Radiol 2013;23(4):931–7.

13. Seraj SM, Zadeh MZ, Werner T, et al. O4: 03 PM Abstract No. 235 Pre-treatment FDG-PET can predict the survival after Yttrium-90 radio-embolization in metastatic liver disease. J Vasc Interv Radiol 2019;30(3):S105–6.

14. Park S, Kim T-S, Kang SH, et al. 11C-acetate and 18F-fluorodeoxyglucose positron emission tomography/computed tomography dual imaging for the prediction of response and prognosis after transarterial chemoembolization. Medicine (Baltimore) 2018;97(37):e12311.

15. Piduru SM, Schuster DM, Barron BJ, et al. Prognostic value of 18F-fluorodeoxyglucose positron emission tomography–computed tomography in predicting survival in patients with unresectable metastatic melanoma to the liver undergoing yttrium-90 radioembolization. J Vasc Interv Radiol 2012;23(7):943–8.

16. Jreige M, Mitsakis P, Van Der Gucht A, et al. 18 F-FDG PET/CT predicts survival after 90 Y transarterial radioembolization in unresectable hepatocellular carcinoma. Eur J Nucl Med Mol Imaging 2017;44(7):1215–22.

17. Kim MJ, Kim YS, Cho YH, et al. Use of 18F-FDG PET to predict tumor progression and survival in patients with intermediate hepatocellular carcinoma treated by transarterial chemoembolization. Korean J Intern Med 2015;30(3):308.

18. Lee JW, Oh JK, Chung YA, et al. Prognostic significance of 18F-FDG uptake in hepatocellular carcinoma treated with transarterial chemoembolization or concurrent chemoradiotherapy: a multicenter retrospective cohort study. J Nucl Med 2016;57(4):509–16.

19. Joosten J, Jager G, Oyen W, et al. Cryosurgery and radiofrequency ablation for unresectable colorectal liver metastases. Eur J Surg Oncol 2005;31(10):1152–9.

20. Langenhoff B, Oyen W, Jager G, et al. Efficacy of fluorine-18-deoxyglucose positron emission tomography in detecting tumor recurrence after local ablative therapy for liver metastases: a prospective study. J Clin Oncol 2002;20(22):4453–8.

21. Hayden MR, Tyagi SC, Kolb L, et al. Vascular ossification–calcification in metabolic syndrome, type 2 diabetes mellitus, chronic kidney disease, and calciphylaxis–calcific uremic arteriolopathy: the emerging role of sodium thiosulfate. Cardiovasc Diabetol 2005;4(1):4.

22. Michl M, Lehner S, Paprottka PM, et al. Use of PERCIST for prediction of progression-free and overall survival after radioembolization for liver metastases from pancreatic cancer. J Nucl Med 2016;57(3):355–60.

23. Shady W, Kishore S, Gavane S, et al. Metabolic tumor volume and total lesion glycolysis on FDG-PET/CT can predict overall survival after 90Y radioembolization of colorectal liver metastases: a

comparison with SUVmax, SUVpeak, and RECIST 1.0. Eur J Radiol 2016;85(6):1224–31.

24. Fendler WP, Tiega DBP, Ilhan H, et al. Validation of several SUV-based parameters derived from 18F-FDG PET for prediction of survival after SIRT of hepatic metastases from colorectal cancer. J Nucl Med 2013;54(8):1202–8.

25. Ziai P, Hayeri MR, Salei A, et al. Role of optimal quantification of FDG PET imaging in the clinical practice of radiology. Radiographics 2016;36(2):481–96.

26. Taghvaei R, Zadeh MZ, Sirous R, et al. Pre-treatment partial-volume-corrected TLG is the best predictor of overall survival in patients with relapsing/refractory non-hodgkin lymphoma following radioimmunotherapy. Am J Nucl Med Mol Imaging 2018;8(6):407.

27. Alavi A, Werner TJ, Høilund-Carlsen PF, et al. Correction for partial volume effect is a must, not a luxury, to fully exploit the potential of quantitative PET imaging in clinical oncology. Mol Imaging Biol 2018;20(1):1–3.

28. Torigian DA, Lopez R, Alapati S, et al. Feasibility and performance of novel software to quantify metabolically active volumes and 3D partial volume corrected SUV and metabolic volumetric products of spinal bone marrow metastases on 18F-FDG-PET/CT. Hell J Nucl Med 2011;14(1):8–14.

29. Roh JL, Kim JS, Kang BC, et al. Clinical significance of pretreatment metabolic tumor volume and total lesion glycolysis in hypopharyngeal squamous cell carcinomas. J Surg Oncol 2014;110(7):869–75.

30. Lee SM, Bae SK, Kim TH, et al. Value of 18F-FDG PET/CT for early prediction of pathologic response (by residual cancer burden criteria) of locally advanced breast cancer to neoadjuvant chemotherapy. Clin Nucl Med 2014;39(10):882–6.

31. Salavati A, Duan F, Snyder BS, et al. Optimal FDG PET/CT volumetric parameters for risk stratification in patients with locally advanced non-small cell lung cancer: results from the ACRIN 6668/RTOG 0235 trial. Eur J Nucl Med Mol Imaging 2017;44(12):1969–83.

32. Zhuang H, Pourdehnad M, Lambright ES, et al. Dual time point 18F-FDG PET imaging for differentiating malignant from inflammatory processes. J Nucl Med 2001;42(9):1412–7.

33. Matthies A, Hickeson M, Cuchiara A, et al. Dual time point 18F-FDG PET for the evaluation of pulmonary nodules. J Nucl Med 2002;43(7):871–5.

34. Hamberg LM, Hunter GJ, Alpert NM, et al. The dose uptake ratio as an index of glucose metabolism:

useful parameter or oversimplification? J Nucl Med 1994;35(8):1308–12.

35. Lodge MA, Lucas JD, Marsden PK, et al. A PET study of 18 FDG uptake in soft tissue masses. Eur J Nucl Med 1999;26(1):22–30.

36. Hustinx R, Smith RJ, Benard F, et al. Dual time point fluorine-18 fluorodeoxyglucose positron emission tomography: a potential method to differentiate malignancy from inflammation and normal tissue in the head and neck. Eur J Nucl Med 1999;26(10):1345–8.

37. Wu B, Zhao Y, Zhang Y, et al. Does dual-time-point 18F-FDG PET/CT scan add in the diagnosis of hepatocellular carcinoma? Hell J Nucl Med 2017;20(1):79–82.

38. Koyama K, Okamura T, Kawabe J, et al. The usefulness of 18 F-FDG PET images obtained 2 hours after intravenous injection in liver tumor. Ann Nucl Med 2002;16(3):169.

39. Fuster D, Lafuente S, Setoain X, et al. Dual-time point images of the liver with 18F-FDG PET/CT in suspected recurrence from colorectal cancer. Rev Esp Med Nucl Imagen Mol 2012;31(3):111–6.

40. Cheng G, Alavi A, Lim E, et al. Dynamic changes of FDG uptake and clearance in normal tissues. Mol Imaging Biol 2013;15(3):345–52.

41. Seraj SM, Al-Zaghal A, Zadeh MZ, et al. Dynamics of fluorine-18-fluorodeoxyglucose uptake in the liver and its correlation with hepatic fat content and BMI. Nucl Med Commun 2019;40(5):545–51.

42. Kubota K, Itoh M, Ozaki K, et al. Advantage of delayed whole-body FDG-PET imaging for tumour detection. Eur J Nucl Med 2001;28(6):696–703.

43. Nishiyama Y, Yamamoto Y, Monden T, et al. Evaluation of delayed additional FDG PET imaging in patients with pancreatic tumour. Nucl Med Commun 2005;26(10):895–901.

44. Chirindel A, Alluri K, Tahari AK, et al. Liver SULmean at FDG PET/CT: effect of FDG uptake time. Clin Nucl Med 2015;40(1):e17.

45. Dirisamer A, Halpern BS, Schima W, et al. Dual-time-point FDG-PET/CT for the detection of hepatic metastases. Mol Imaging Biol 2008;10(6):335–40.

46. Chan WL, Ramsay SC, Szeto ER, et al. Dual-time-point 18F-FDG-PET/CT imaging in the assessment of suspected malignancy. J Med Imaging Radiat Oncol 2011;55(4):379–90.

47. Taghvaei R, Oestergaard B, Zadeh MZ, et al. Correlation of dual time point FDG-PET with response to chemotherapy in multiple myeloma. J Nucl Med 2017;58(supplement 1):188.

Fluorodeoxyglucose-PET for Ablation Treatment Planning, Intraprocedural Monitoring, and Response

Sirish A. Kishore, MD[a], Michael J. Drabkin, MD[b,1],
Constantinos T. Sofocleous, MD, PhD, FSIR, FCIRSE[a,*]

KEYWORDS

- PET scan • Positron-emission tomography • Biopsy • Ablation • Interventional radiology
- Radiology • Interventional oncology

KEY POINTS

- PET has become an essential tool for staging and response assessment in oncologic imaging.
- Real-time image guidance in PET/computed tomography (CT) scanners for interventional procedures decreases the misregistration and image compatibility issues that limit fusion software.
- PET/CT-guided biopsies have greater sensitivity and diagnostic yield for fluorodeoxyglucose-avid lesions, particularly those that are poorly delineated on standard anatomic imaging modalities.
- The split-dose technique for PET-guided ablation offers the potential for the immediate identification and reablation of metabolically active residual viable tumor.
- PET has the potential to be a major tool for image-guided minimally invasive therapy and more broadly for personalized medicine as a whole.

BACKGROUND

Innovation in minimally invasive technology, together with advances in imaging, allows interventional radiology to provide superior precision in image-guided diagnosis and treatment, while also decreasing periprocedural morbidity.[1] Molecular imaging provides physiologic metabolic information that, combined with anatomic localization, has unique potential to further enhance the capabilities of image-guided interventions. PET in particular, allows for improved spatial resolution as well as the acquisition of quantitative data in comparison to other molecular imaging techniques. PET has become an essential tool for staging and response assessment in oncologic imaging. It is commonly used in conjunction with computed tomography (CT) (PET/CT), and less frequently MR imaging (PET/MR imaging), as a hybrid imaging modality. Over the past decade it has also evolved into a tool for image-guided interventions, specifically in the rapidly growing field of interventional oncology. This review discusses the current and evolving role of metabolic imaging, specifically PET, in interventional oncology.

PET-GUIDED PERCUTANEOUS BIOPSY AND ABLATION

Because of the spatial resolution and specificity of lesion identification afforded by PET, both biopsy (**Fig. 1**) and ablation (**Figs. 2** and **3**) have been early

Disclosures: None (S. Kishore, M.J. Drabkin). Research Support: BTG, Ethicon J&J, Consultant: Ethicon J&J, Terumo, GE (C.T. Sofocleous).
[a] Interventional Radiology Service, Memorial Sloan Kettering Cancer, 1275 York, IR Suite H118, New York City, NY 10065, USA; [b] Interventional Radiology Service, Memorial Sloan Kettering Cancer, New York City, NY, USA
[1] Present address: 39 Barberry Lane, Roslyn Heights, NY 11577.
* Corresponding author.
E-mail address: sofoclec@mskcc.org

PET Clin 14 (2019) 427–436
https://doi.org/10.1016/j.cpet.2019.06.006

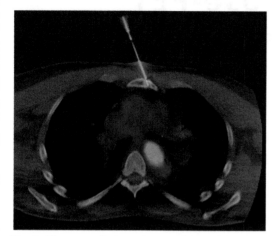

Fig. 1. Biopsy needle in an FDG-avid sternal lesion on PET-CT.

applications of PET technology in interventional oncology. This is often achieved through image registration using preprocedure PET images and navigation systems and rarely with real-time image guidance in dedicated PET/CT imaging suites.[2–5] Real-time image guidance in PET/CT scanners for interventional procedures decreases the misregistration and image compatibility issues that limit fusion software. Although any PET/CT can be used for interventions, there are certain requirements that facilitate this application, which include the availability of trained staff able to provide support during invasive procedures and image acquisition, as well as rooms that provide space and gas lines for anesthesia. In-room image display is preferable, and large bore scanners are needed to accommodate both patients and interventional equipment in the gantry.[6] The use of anesthesia for deep sedation and capabilities of general anesthesia with paralysis and respiratory control are useful. This allows for breath-hold image acquisition protocols to decrease or even eliminate misregistration and breathing artifacts. Without anesthesia, these artifacts can be problematic for real-time PET image acquisition, particularly for tumors located near the diaphragm.[3,7] Radiotracer dose administration and relevant workflow considerations need be tailored to the specific intervention of interest and will be discussed herein.

PET-Guided Biopsy

Percutaneous biopsy is a critical component of cancer care. Improved mechanisms of tissue acquisition and the sophistication of subsequent tissue analysis enhance initial diagnosis, response to therapy assessment, and decision-making. Although targeted percutaneous biopsy is typically

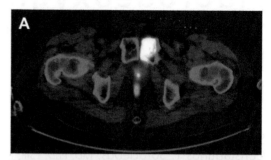

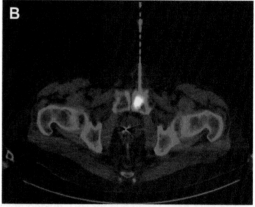

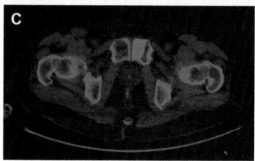

Fig. 2. (*A*) PET-CT demonstrating FDG-avid left pubic lesion. (*B*) Cryoablation probe seen within the lesion. (*C*) Postablation PET-CT demonstrates near-complete resolution of previously noted PET activity within the lesion.

performed with simple CT or ultrasound guidance, PET/CT-guided biopsies have greater sensitivity and diagnostic yield for fluorodeoxyglucose (FDG)-avid lesions, particularly those that are poorly delineated on standard anatomic imaging modalities.[8–10] In addition, in the absence of clear morphologic features on anatomic imaging, PET can facilitate the identification of viable disease within areas of necrosis or intermixed with adjacent reactive or inflammatory changes. This is particularly useful when evaluating large complex masses with internal necrosis or in the lung where the distinction between malignancy and atelectasis or consolidation can be limited when relying

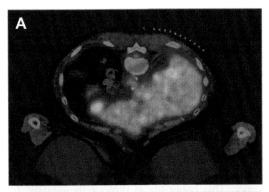

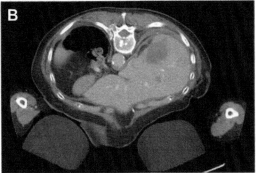

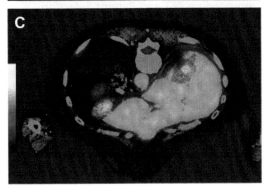

Fig. 3. (A) PET-CT demonstrating FDG-avid lesion in right posterior liver. (B) Portal venous phase postablation CT demonstrates ablation zone. (C) Fusion of (A) and (B) shows that the original lesion is within the ablation zone as well as an appropriate ablation margin (>5 mm).

on conventional anatomic imaging alone.[11,12] Postprocedural analysis of specimens obtained under PET guidance can also provide confirmation of adequate tissue sampling via autoradiographic techniques. Using image coregistration, PET can confirm that both the sampling location and acquired material are sufficient for advanced molecular analyses and radiogenomics.[13,14] Scintigraphic thresholds can also be used to determine the adequacy and accuracy of percutaneous biopsy for image-tissue correlation. Examination of the biopsy specimen with a scintillation counter can confirm that the sampled region is in fact FDG-avid. This may be of particular importance in confirming adequate tissue sampling when the biopsy is found to be benign on the pathology report.

PET imaging can provide important insights into biological processes at the cellular level. Identification of a target with the greatest glycolytic activity amongst multiple sites of FDG avidity can direct tissue sampling to the areas of greatest clinical importance. This enables targeting of the highest grade disease or cell populations refractory to therapy based on established diagnostic PET imaging criteria.[15,16] This information may also have important implications for staging. In lymphoma, for example, nontargeted iliac crest biopsy is performed to evaluate bone marrow involvement; PET/CT-guided bone marrow biopsy may allow for superior accuracy in patients with focal marrow findings on prebiopsy PET/CT.[17]

The development of new tracers has allowed patients with a wide variety of disease processes to benefit from PET-guided tissue sampling. For example, tracers directed toward prostate-specific membrane antigen not only enhance lesion identification but also may be crucial for the detection of viable cancer cells in tumors that are not consistently FDG-avid.[18,19] Different PET tracers can also be used to demonstrate divergent tumor biology within the same index lesion. Tissue sampling under PET guidance in such tumors can detect clonal subpopulations through targeting of areas of differential radiotracer uptake as needed.[20,21] As an increasing number of radiotracers become clinically available for diagnosis, PET-guided biopsy offers validation of these probes as in vivo surrogate biomarkers. These radiotracers can then be used directly in image-guided intervention. This gives PET tremendous potential for an expanded role in the era of personalized medicine.

PET-Guided Ablation

Real-time PET imaging can provide valuable image guidance during therapeutic minimally invasive procedures. Similar to biopsy, intraprocedural PET can aid in accurate needle placement for ablation of PET-avid tumors minimizing the number of needle passes. More importantly, PET/CT can be used to assess tumor response after ablation.[22] However, attempts to use FDG-PET intraprocedurally and immediately postablation have had challenges. FDG-PET/CT imaging within 24 hours of ablation is generally obscured by reactive inflammation that limits the ability to detect residual viable tumor within the ablation zone (AZ).[23]

There is often morphologic distortion immediately postablation without significant change in overall FDG avidity, hindering the assessment of tumor destruction during ablation.[24] At the authors' institution postablation venous phase CT imaging is fused with preprocedure PET images in order to delineate the AZ for liver lesions (see **Fig. 3**).

Recently nitrogen 13 ammonia perfusion PET has been used for AZ evaluation.[25] The combination of preablation metabolic imaging and immediate postablation imaging with ammonia perfusion PET/CT has been shown to effectively delineate the margins of the AZ, which can be measured against the margins of the original lesion.[25] However, this is likely less helpful than direct assessment of residual metabolically active disease as is possible with FDG-PET.

The split-dose technique is used as a strategy that allows targeting and immediate postablation assessment of treatment completeness or residual viable tissue within the AZ.[2] This involves the administration of 2 different doses of FDG, one before and one immediately after the ablation.[2] The conventional 444 MBq FDG dose for diagnostic PET/CT is divided into 2 doses: initially a 148 MBq dose is administered within 1 hour before ablation to delineate the tumor and aid guidance of probe/electrode placement. Second, a 296 MBq FDG dose is administered once the ablation is completed; this allows for immediate assessment of the AZ. The smaller first dose decays over time and is dwarfed by the larger second dose (administered 2 to 3 hours later), allowing for adequate visualization of FDG activity in any residual viable tumor. It should be noted that with this method the ablated tumor may still have minimal activity in the immediate postablation period in the absence of residual viable disease originating from the initial preablation dose (see **Fig. 2**C). A qualitative assessment of the postablation PET/CT can be performed by identifying the presence and pattern of FDG activity within the AZ and surrounding parenchyma. The Tissue Radioactivity Concentration (TRC) ratio serves as a quantitative measure: TRC ratio = [(Lesion TRCmax–Liver TRCmean)/Lesion TRCmax] x 100.[26]

Immediate postablation PET/CT using the split-dose technique has been shown to be an effective early indicator of treatment success.[27] Using Receiver Operating Characteristic curve analysis, a TRC ratio of greater than 28.3 in the treatment zone had a 100% positive predictive value for detecting residual disease and was superior to contrast-enhanced CT.[27] These imaging observations were confirmed with postprocedural biopsies of the AZ in patients with colorectal metastasis to the liver. As expected, there was a strong correlation between greater standardized uptake value (SUV) and a positive tumor biopsy result.[28] The SUV ratio (calculated as the SUV of the AZ divided by the pretreatment SUV of the tumor) and minimum ablation margin (MM < 5 mm as assessed on dynamic CT) were independent predictors of local recurrence in those patients with negative AZ biopsies immediately postablation (median follow-up of 22.5 months).[29] The split-dose technique for PET-guided ablation offers the potential for the immediate identification and reablation of metabolically active residual viable tumor. This capability is profoundly valuable for optimizing image-guided tumor ablation as a local cancer cure.

PET AND TRANSARTERIAL THERAPIES

PET can also be used in conjunction with transarterial therapy to aid in patient selection, dosimetric assessment for treatment radioisotope administration (ie, Yttrium-90 [Y90]), and treatment response for a variety of tumor pathologies and treatment modalities.[30–32]

Preprocedure PET and Patient Selection

FDG-PET, together with standard morphologic imaging, can be used for detection and staging. It also carries additional value as a means of response assessment following intraarterial therapy of FDG-avid liver tumors. Preprocedure FDG-PET biomarkers have been shown to predict response to transarterial therapies.[33] The quantitative nature of PET allows for multidimensional volumetric metabolic tumor assessment. In patients undergoing transarterial chemoembolization (TACE) or transarterial chemoinfusion for hepatocellular carcinoma (HCC), metabolic tumor volume (MTV) on pretreatment PET/CT was an independent predictor of progression-free survival (PFS) and overall survival (OS). Specifically a greater MTV was associated with a worse prognosis.[34] MTV is defined as the sum of lesional voxels greater than the 97.5th percentile of normal liver voxels. In another series of patients undergoing transarterial radioembolization for unresectable HCC, the tumor-to-liver uptake ratio and SUVmax (the most avid voxel within a region of interest) were independent negative predictors of PFS and OS.[35] These observations, in conjunction with advanced computational methods, elucidate more sophisticated PET-based radiomic signatures that are of pretreatment prognostic value.[36]

Preembolotherapy PET can also have predictive value for tumors that do not consistently demonstrate increased glycolysis, such as HCC. C11-acetate PET reflects increased cell membrane synthesis in tumor tissue and may predict HCC response to transarterial therapy, particularly as part of a dual-tracer imaging protocol with FDG.[37,38] In patients undergoing TACE, dual-tracer PET/CT demonstrated differential risk stratification and prognosis based on staging. The tumor-to-liver FDG-uptake ratio was an independent predictor of recurrence in intermediate stage patients. In advanced stage patients, only the dual-tracer uptake ratio of FDG to acetate independently predicted recurrence.[38] Another study assessed effective radioembolization dosimetry stratified by preprocedure dual-tracer PET imaging with C-acetate and FDG as a noninvasive indicator of tumor differentiation. This study found that the absorbed dose-response thresholds varied significantly between poorly differentiated and well or moderately differentiated tumors (262 Gy vs 152 and 174 Gy, respectively). This suggests that stratification using preprocedure multitracer imaging protocols may be useful in personalizing transarterial therapies.[37] Because more molecular imaging agents are validated with histologic assessment and correlation with tumor biology, preprocedure PET imaging may ultimately be used to match those patients with specific tumor phenotypes that are likely to respond to a certain locoregional treatment.

PET-Based Dosimetry Assessment After Y90 Administration

Imaging of Y90 microsphere delivery is possible with both SPECT-CT and PET/CT, depicting Bremsstrahlung radiation and positron emission from Y90, respectively.[39] Although both molecular imaging studies can be used as confirmation of dose delivery and distribution after treatment, posttreatment PET/CT can additionally independently predict treatment efficacy. This is possible because the level of avidity reflects the level of absorbed tumor dose and can be used to generate 3-dimensional (3D) absorbed dose maps aiding in our understanding of dose-based response.[39,40] Dosimetric assessments on pretreatment Tc99m-MAASPECT and posttreatment single-photon emission computed tomography (SPECT) can also be used to predict absorbed tumor dose; however, correlation of calculated absorbed dose to tumor dose on SPECT is much more variable as compared with posttreatment Y90 PET/CT.[39] This could justify a paradigm shift toward utilization of immediate postprocedure PET/CT as a quantitative, and potentially more accurate, predictor of dose delivery to tumor. This would also allow for subsequent correlations to be made between absorbed tumor dose and

response.[41] With appropriate postprocessing, posttreatment Y90 PET/CT can be obtained with acquisition times similar to SPECT-CT and with superior image quality. For all these reasons, PET will likely take an increased role in the assessment of patients undergoing radioembolization.[42]

PET and Assessment of Treatment Response After Transarterial Therapy

Use of tumor volume and dimensions as a means of assessing tumor response after locoregional therapies is problematic. RECIST has been identified as insufficient in the assessment of liver tumors and in particular colon cancer hepatic metastases after treatment.[43] With the increased availability of PET/CT, response criteria for solid tumors have continued to evolve from tumor dimensional size measurements using morphologic imaging to the incorporation of metabolic response criteria. In addition, metabolic imaging allows assessment of tumor glycolysis, a quantitative measure of growth and mitogenesis independent of size.[44,45]

Although formal metabolic response criteria described by PERCIST (PET Response Criteria in Solid Tumors) and EORTC (European Organization for Research and Treatment of Cancer) can provide structured PET response criteria for locoregional therapy, the quantitative nature and spatial resolution of PET in conjunction with advanced postprocessing software has allowed for the development of additional PET biomarkers that can specifically assess response and guide prognosis after locoregional therapy.[46,47] Metrics of FDG-avidity are most commonly based on the SUV, which normalize uptake based on body surface area or lean body mass. These metrics are typically reported as SUVmean (average uptake within a region of interest), SUVmax, and SUVpeak (the maximum average uptake within a voxel). SUVpeak has been shown to demonstrate the least variability in tumors with variable acquisition time.[48]

Volumetric PET metrics can also provide valuable information about the metabolic phenotype of a tumor, reflecting both size and extent of metabolic activity. Two such metrics are MTV, or the entire 3D volume of tumor that is FDG-avid, and total lesion glycolysis (TLG), which is SUVmean multiplied by the MTV.[47] Not only can these volumetric measures provide risk stratification across a variety of solid tumor types, but TLG is also supported by PERCIST as an optional measure to assess metabolically active tumor burden (although not formally part of PERCIST criteria).[47]

In assessing early response to radioembolization (which can take several months to manifest by standard size and density criteria on anatomic imaging), change in SUVmax between preprocedure and 6 to 8 weeks post-PET/CT was significantly correlated with changes in serum tumor markers and strongly predicted PFS in patients undergoing radioembolization for liver-dominant metastatic colorectal cancer. Tumor density and RECIST criteria on anatomic imaging did not predict PFS in these patients.[49]

Volumetric PET measures may also provide improved and earlier prognostic information after radioembolization. A comparison between TLG on PET/CT and longest tumor diameter (LTD) on MR imaging for liver-predominant colorectal liver metastases found that both predicted OS at 3 months. TLG was also able to predict OS at 1 month, and more importantly LTD may have actually underestimated responders (as identified by TLG criteria). This suggests that TLG, in addition to providing an objective and replicable semi-automated quantitative biomarker, may be more accurate and sensitive in determining response and prognosis after radioembolization and at an earlier time point posttreatment than RECIST.[50] A comparison between the metrics of FDG avidity (SUVmean, SUVmax, SUVpeak, MTV, and TLG) and RECIST in assessing OS of patients undergoing radioembolization for colorectal liver metastases found that MTV and TLG were the only significant predictors of OS after radioembolization. These findings further support that RECIST is not useful and that metabolic imaging and, in particular, volumetric PET/CT can be valuable predictors of response to hepatic-directed locoregional therapies such as radioembolization.[46]

The use of PET allows for earlier and more sensitive detection of recurrent disease following both arterial therapy and ablation. The implementation of non-FDG radiotracers will further improve the specificity of metabolic imaging, with disease-specific probes that may allow tailored assessments and interventions based on specific disease processes.[51–54]

WORKFLOW CONSIDERATIONS

Safe and effective use of PET/CT suites for image-guided procedures requires that certain measures be taken in order to optimize workflow and to ensure quality and safety.

Radiotracer Timing and Dose

The dose and timing of radiotracer administration are important for PET-guided biopsy and ablation protocols to ensure sufficient time for radiotracer accumulation at the target while maintaining safe levels of exposure to operating physicians and

staff. Personnel safety guidelines have been previously established.[55] At the authors' institution, 222 MBq of FDG is administered for PET-guided biopsies approximately 30 to 45 minutes before the procedure. For ablation using the split-dose method, approximately 148 MBq of FDG is administered before the procedure, and another 296 MBq is administered after completion of the ablation. Imaging obtained intraprocedurally is typically performed 30 to 60 minutes after each injection. FDG has a half-life of 110 minutes that could potentially pose problems for shorter ablations when the first dose has not had sufficient time to decay before postablation imaging. This, however, is unlikely to be an issue in current clinical practice. For shorter procedures this issue could be circumvented with the advent of new and emerging radionuclides that have shorter half-lives.

Staffing and Perioperative Considerations

To effectively use PET for interventions it is necessary to have a well-trained staff.[56] Intraprocedural imaging is performed by technologists trained in PET and who often undergo additional training in interventional radiology so that they are able to understand the technical aspects of image-guided needle localization. In the perioperative setting, nurses should be aware of the radiation risks associated with radiotracer administration and trained on appropriate safety precautions. At the authors' institution, they have dedicated rooms for patients undergoing PET-guided procedures. These are used for preprocedure assessment and postoperative recovery (Fig. 4). PET-guided procedures require substantial additional preoperative time and resources, given the time it takes for radiotracer accumulation for imaging before the procedure. In the perioperative period, it is critical to convey precautionary information to family and staff about exposure, as radiation dose is primarily related to proximity to the patient.[55]

For the operator and procedural staff, the procedural exposure is not significantly different than that of standard fluoroscopic procedures. However, given that the 511 keV photon from PET is higher energy than the typical x-ray photon, standard protective equipment (ie, lead) is not effective against radiation from PET-guided procedures.[55] The median effective dose for a PET-guided ablation is 0.02 mSV to the operator, 0.01 mSV to the anesthesiologist, and 0.02 mSV to the technologist.[55] Radiopharmaceutical doses in the protocols were reduced (relative to diagnostic PET/CT) in order to minimize dose to the procedural personnel while at the same time maintaining image quality.

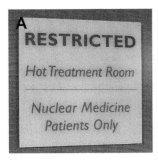 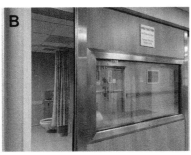

Fig. 4. (A) Sign indicating a restricted hot treatment room. (B) Hot room for patients to recover after radionuclide injection. A closing door minimizes accidental entry and dampens radiation to passersby. A personal toilet helps minimize the risk of the affected patient's bodily fluids coming into contact with others.

Cost-Effectiveness

Although PET-guided interventions are safe and effective, their ultimate application hinges on cost-effectiveness, as these procedures generally require staff with additional training, additional periprocedural and intraprocedural time, dedicated PET scanner time, as well as provisions for rooms with enough space for interventions and gas lines for anesthesia. If cases are appropriately selected, these costs should be offset by improved diagnostic biopsy yield and by increased ablation effectiveness. This translates into fewer repeat treatments and earlier assessment of treatment response and prognosis in patients undergoing interventional therapy.

PET-scanners are available in most large medical centers in the United States. Given that the most of the procedures requiring PET guidance are elective, PET scanners can be used as needed for interventions without significantly affecting the diagnostic workflow provided that there is appropriate planning and staffing in place.

FUTURE DIRECTIONS

The authors expect that PET will continue to gain an increased role in interventional radiology and specifically interventional oncology. It has the potential to be a major tool for image-guided minimally invasive therapy and more broadly for personalized medicine as a whole. Novel radiotracers continue to emerge, and physicians are becoming progressively more comfortable incorporating PET into interventional therapy. As the development of molecular imaging continues to parallel advances in the understanding of molecular mechanisms in cancer, the interface of PET and interventional radiology will continue to grow, both for tissue sampling and treatment.

The increasing use of PET in the assessment of therapeutic response results in earlier identification of disease that is amenable to image-guided therapies such as PET-guided ablation. These developments can help to minimize chemotherapy exposure and associated toxicity. They also allow for early minimally invasive treatment of refractory disease, potentially allowing for eradication of the refractory clonal cell lines.

Increased sophistication of PET imaging, computing technology, and data science may allow for earlier triage to locoregional therapies as our understanding continues to evolve and as we begin to understand the radiomic signatures that affect outcome. Finally, PET-based dosimetry will likely further expand and hopefully optimize the administration of internal radiation therapies such as intra-arterial radioembolization with microspheres.[57]

REFERENCES

1. Smith KA, Kim HS. Interventional radiology and image-guided medicine: interventional oncology. SeminOncol 2011;38(1):151–62.
2. Ryan ER, Sofocleous CT, Schöder H, et al. Split-dose technique for FDG PET/CT-guided percutaneous ablation: a method to facilitate lesion targeting and to provide immediate assessment of treatment effectiveness. Radiology 2013;268(1):288–95.
3. Shyn PB, Tatli S, Sahni VA, et al. PET/CT-guided percutaneous liver mass biopsies and ablations: targeting accuracy of a single 20 s breath-hold PET acquisition. ClinRadiol 2014;69(4):410–5.
4. Tatli S, Gerbaudo VH, Mamede M, et al. Abdominal masses sampled at PET/CT-guided percutaneous biopsy: initial experience with registration of prior PET/CT images. Radiology 2010;256(1):305–11.
5. Venkatesan AM, Kadoury S, Abi-Jaoudeh N, et al. Real-time FDG PET guidance during biopsies and radiofrequency ablation using multimodality fusion with electromagnetic navigation. Radiology 2011; 260(3):848–56.
6. Solomon SB, Cornelis F. Interventional molecular imaging. J Nucl Med 2016;57(4):493–6.
7. Li G, Schmidtlein CR, Burger IA, et al. Assessing and accounting for the impact of respiratory motion on FDG uptake and viable volume for liver lesions in free-breathing PET using respiration-suspended

PET images as reference. Med Phys 2014;41(9): 091905.

8. Cerci JJ, Tabacchi E, Bogoni M. Fluorodeoxyglucose-PET/computed tomography-guided biopsy. PET Clin 2016;11(1):57–64.

9. Cornelis F, Silk M, Schoder H, et al. Performance of intra-procedural 18-fluorodeoxyglucose PET/CT-guided biopsies for lesions suspected of malignancy but poorly visualized with other modalities. Eur J Nucl Med MolImaging 2014;41(12):2265–72.

10. Paparo F, Piccazzo R, Cevasco L, et al. Advantages of percutaneous abdominal biopsy under PET-CT/ultrasound fusion imaging guidance: a pictorial essay. AbdomImaging 2014;39(5):1102–13.

11. Guralnik L, Rozenberg R, Frenkel A, et al. Metabolic PET/CT-guided lung lesion biopsies: impact on diagnostic accuracy and rate of sampling error. J Nucl Med 2015;56(4):518–22.

12. Radhakrishnan RK, Mittal BR, Gorla AKR, et al. Real-time intraprocedural18F-FDG PET/CT-guided biopsy using automated robopsy arm (ARA) in the diagnostic evaluation of thoracic lesions with prior inconclusive biopsy results: initial experience from a tertiary health care centre. Br J Radiol 2017; 90(1080):20170258.

13. Fanchon LM, Dogan S, Moreira AL, et al. Feasibility of in situ, high-resolution correlation of tracer uptake with histopathology by quantitative autoradiography of biopsy specimens obtained under 18F-FDG PET/CT guidance. J Nucl Med 2015;56(4): 538–44.

14. Kirov AS, Fanchon LM, Seiter D, et al. Technical Note: scintillation well counters and particle counting digital autoradiography devices can be used to detect activities associated with genomic profiling adequacy of biopsy specimens obtained after a low activity 18 F-FDG injection. Med Phys 2018; 45(5):2179–85.

15. Chirindel A, Chaudhry M, Blakeley JO, et al. 18F-FDG PET/CT qualitative and quantitative evaluation in neurofibromatosis type 1 patients for detection of malignant transformation: comparison of early to delayed imaging with and without liver activity normalization. J Nucl Med 2015;56(3):379–85.

16. Karls S, Shah H, Jacene H. PET/CT for lymphoma post-therapy response assessment in other lymphomas, response assessment for autologous stem cell transplant, and lymphoma follow-up. SeminNucl Med 2018;48(1):37–49.

17. Hao B, Zhao L, Luo N-N, et al. Is it sufficient to evaluate bone marrow involvement in newly diagnosed lymphomas using 18F-FDG PET/CT and/or routine iliac crest biopsy? A new approach of PET/CT-guided targeted bone marrow biopsy. BMC Cancer 2018;18(1):1192.

18. Rowe SP, Macura KJ, Mena E, et al. PSMA-based [(18)F]DCFPyL PET/CT is superior to conventional imaging for lesion detection in patients with metastatic prostate cancer. MolImaging Biol 2016;18(3): 411–9.

19. Rowe SP, Gorin MA, Hammers HJ, et al. Detection of 18F-FDG PET/CT occult lesions with 18F-DCFPyL PET/CT in a patient with metastatic renal cell carcinoma. ClinNucl Med 2016;41(1):83–5.

20. Ulaner GA, Goldman DA, Gönen M, et al. Initial results of a prospective clinical trial of 18F-fluciclovine PET/CT in newly diagnosed invasive ductal and invasive lobular breast cancers. J Nucl Med 2016; 57(9):1350–6.

21. Cornelis FH, Durack JC, Morris MJ, et al. Effective prostate-specific membrane antigen-based 18F-DCFPyL-guided cryoablation of a single positive site in a patient believed to be more metastatic on 11C-choline PET/CT. ClinNucl Med 2017;42(12): e516–8.

22. McLoney ED, Isaacson AJ, Keating P. The role of PET imaging before, during, and after percutaneous hepatic and pulmonary tumor ablation. SeminInterv-Radiol 2014;31(2):187–92.

23. Vandenbroucke F, Vandemeulebroucke J, Ilsen B, et al. Predictive value of pattern classification 24 hours after radiofrequency ablation of liver metastases on CT and positron emission tomography/CT. J VascIntervRadiol 2014;25(8):1240–9.

24. Schoellnast H, Larson SM, Nehmeh SA, et al. Radiofrequency ablation of non-small-cell carcinoma of the lung under real-time FDG PET CT guidance. CardiovascInterventRadiol 2011;34(Suppl2):S182–5.

25. Shyn PB, Casadaban LC, Sainani NI, et al. Intraprocedural ablation margin assessment by using ammonia perfusion PET during FDG PET/CT-guided liver tumor ablation: a pilot study. Radiology 2018;288(1): 138–45.

26. Keiding S. Bringing physiology into PET of the liver. J Nucl Med 2012;53(3):425–33.

27. Cornelis F, Sotirchos V, Violari E, et al. 18F-FDG PET/CT is an immediate imaging biomarker of treatment success after liver metastasis ablation. J Nucl Med 2016;57(7):1052–7.

28. Sotirchos VS, Petrovic LM, Gönen M, et al. Colorectal cancer liver metastases: biopsy of the ablation zone and margins can be used to predict oncologic outcome. Radiology 2016;280(3): 949–59.

29. Cornelis FH, Petre EN, Vakiani E, et al. Immediate postablation18F-FDG injection and corresponding SUV are surrogate biomarkers of local tumor progression after thermal ablation of colorectal carcinoma liver metastases. J Nucl Med 2018;59(9): 1360–5.

30. Eaton BR, Kim HS, Schreibmann E, et al. Quantitative dosimetry for yttrium-90 radionuclide therapy: tumor dose predicts fluorodeoxyglucose positron emission tomography response in hepatic

metastatic melanoma. J VascIntervRadiol 2014; 25(2):288–95.

31. Mehta R, Cai K, Kumar N, et al. A lesion-based response prediction model using pretherapy PET/CT image features for Y90radioembolization to hepatic malignancies. TechnolCancer Res Treat 2017; 16(5):620–9.

32. Vouche M, Salem R, Miller FH, et al. Y90radioembolization of colorectal cancer liver metastases: response assessment by contrast-enhanced computed tomography with or without PET-CT guidance. ClinImaging 2015;39(3):454–62.

33. Yaprak O, Acar S, Ertugrul G, et al. Role of pre-transplant 18F-FDG PET/CT in predicting hepatocellular carcinoma recurrence after liver transplantation. World J GastrointestOncol 2018;10(10): 336–43.

34. Lee JW, Yun M, Cho A, et al. The predictive value of metabolic tumor volume on FDG PET/CT for transarterial chemoembolization and transarterial chemotherapy infusion in hepatocellular carcinoma patients without extrahepatic metastasis. Ann Nucl Med 2015;29(5):400–8.

35. Jreige M, Mitsakis P, Van Der Gucht A, et al. 18F-FDG PET/CT predicts survival after 90Ytransarterialradioembolization in unresectable hepatocellular carcinoma. Eur J Nucl Med MolImaging 2017; 44(7):1215–22.

36. Blanc-Durand P, Van Der Gucht A, Jreige M, et al. Signature of survival: a 18F-FDG PET based whole-liver radiomic analysis predicts survival after 90Y-TARE for hepatocellular carcinoma. Oncotarget 2018; 9(4):4549–58.

37. Ho CL, Chen S, Cheung SK, et al. Radioembolization with 90Y glass microspheres for hepatocellular carcinoma: significance of pretreatment 11C-acetate and 18F-FDG PET/CT and posttreatment90Y PET/CT in individualized dose prescription. Eur J Nucl Med MolImaging 2018;45(12):2110–21.

38. Park S, Kim T-S, Kang SH, et al. 11C-acetate and 18F-fluorodeoxyglucose positron emission tomography/computed tomography dual imaging for the prediction of response and prognosis after transarterial chemoembolization. Medicine (Baltimore) 2018;97(37): e12311.

39. Pasciak AS, Bourgeois AC, McKinney JM, et al. Radioembolization and the dynamic role of (90)Y PET/CT. Front Oncol 2014;4:38.

40. Song YS, Paeng JC, Kim H-C, et al. PET/CT-Based dosimetry in 90Y-microsphere selective internal radiation therapy: single cohort comparison with pretreatment planning on (99m)Tc-MAA imaging and correlation with treatment efficacy. Medicine (Baltimore) 2015;94(23):e945.

41. Haste P, Tann M, Persohn S, et al. Correlation of technetium-99mmacroaggregatedalbumin and yttrium-90 glass microsphere biodistribution in hepatocellular carcinoma: a retrospective review of pretreatment single photon emission CT and posttreatment positron emission tomography/CT. J VascIntervRadiol 2017;28(5):722–30.e1.

42. Wright CL, Binzel K, Zhang J, et al. Clinical feasibility of 90Y digital PET/CT for imaging microsphere biodistribution following radioembolization. Eur J Nucl Med MolImaging 2017;44(7):1194–7.

43. Janned'Othée B, Sofocleous CT, Hanna N, et al. Development of a research agenda for the management of metastatic colorectal cancer: proceedings from a multidisciplinary research consensus panel. J VascIntervRadiol 2012;23(2):153–63.

44. Pinker K, Riedl C, Weber WA. Evaluating tumor response with FDG PET: updates on PERCIST, comparison with EORTC criteria and clues to future developments. Eur J Nucl Med MolImaging 2017; 44(Suppl 1):55–66.

45. Wahl RL, Jacene H, Kasamon Y, et al. From RECIST to PERCIST: evolving Considerations for PET response criteria in solid tumors. J Nucl Med 2009; 50(Suppl1):122S–1250S.

46. Shady W, Kishore S, Gavane S, et al. Metabolic tumor volume and total lesion glycolysis on FDG-PET/CT can predict overall survival after (90)Y radioembolization of colorectal liver metastases: a comparison with SUVmax, SUVpeak, and RECIST 1.0. Eur J Radiol 2016;85(6):1224–31.

47. Ziai P, Hayeri MR, Salei A, et al. Role of optimal quantification of FDG PET imaging in the clinical practice of radiology. Radiographics 2016;36(2): 481–96.

48. Sher A, Lacoeuille F, Fosse P, et al. For avid glucose tumors, the SUV peak is the most reliable parameter for [(18)F]FDG-PET/CT quantification, regardless of acquisition time. EJNMMI Res 2016;6(1):21.

49. Zerizer I, Al-Nahhas A, Towey D, et al. The role of early 18F-FDG PET/CT in prediction of progression-free survival after 90Yradioembolization: comparison with RECIST and tumour density criteria. Eur J Nucl Med MolImaging 2012;39(9):1391–9.

50. Jongen JMJ, Rosenbaum CENM, Braat MNGJA, et al. Anatomic versus metabolic tumor response assessment after radioembolization treatment. J VascIntervRadiol 2018;29(2):244–53.e2.

51. Packard AT, Broski SM, Callstrom MR, et al. Utility of PET/CT after cryoablation for early identification of local tumor progression in osseous metastatic disease. AJR Am J Roentgenol 2017;208(6):1342–51.

52. Singnurkar A, Solomon SB, Gönen M, et al. 18F-FDG PET/CT for the prediction and detection of local recurrence after radiofrequency ablation of malignant lung lesions. J Nucl Med 2010;51(12):1833–40.

53. Tomasian A, Dehdashti F, Jennings JW. Percutaneous minimally invasive thermal ablation of musculoskeletal lesions: usefulness of PET-computed tomography. PET Clin 2018;13(4):579–85.

54. Cazzato RL, Garnon J, Ramamurthy N, et al. 18F-FDOPA PET/CT-Guided radiofrequency ablation of liver metastases from neuroendocrine tumours: technical note on a preliminary experience. CardiovascInterventRadiol 2016;39(9):1315–21.

55. Ryan ER, Thornton R, Sofocleous CT, et al. PET/CT-guided interventions: personnel radiation dose. CardiovascInterventRadiol 2013;36(4):1063–7.

56. Taylor JS, Keller L, Maybody M. PET/CT-guided interventions in oncology patients: a nursing perspective. J RadiolNurs 2017;36(2):99–103.

57. Kratochwil C, Giesel FL, Bruchertseifer F, et al. [213]Bi-DOTATOC receptor-targeted alpha-radionuclide therapy induces remission in neuroendocrine tumours refractory to beta radiation: a first-in-human experience. Eur J Nucl Med Mollmaging 2014;41(11):2106–19.

Fluorodeoxyglucose PET for Monitoring Response to Embolotherapy (Transarterial Chemoembolization) in Primary and Metastatic Liver Tumors

Isabel Schobert, BS[a,b], Julius Chapiro, MD[a], Darko Pucar, MD, PhD[a],
Lawrence Saperstein, MD[a], Lynn Jeanette Savic, MD[a,b],*

KEYWORDS

- ^{18}F-FDG • PET • TACE • Locoregional therapy • HCC • ICC • mCRC • NET

KEY POINTS

- Transarterial chemoembolization (TACE) is a locoregional treatment of intermediate to advanced stage liver malignancies with combined cytotoxic and ischemic effects.
- Fluorine-18 fluorodeoxyglucose (^{18}F-FDG) PET particularly applied as hybrid imaging with CT or MRI may provide valuable complementary information on treatment efficacy of TACE, as functional alterations in tumor cell metabolism often precede morphologic changes.
- However, ^{18}F-FDG PET is currently merely a niche application for liver cancer imaging and not guideline approved for the clinical management of hepatocellular carcinoma.
- Tumor standard uptake value (SUV) and SUV ratio (tumor$_{max}$/liver$_{mean}$) as well as novel or combined radiotracers may provide quantitative biomarkers for the metabolic activity of liver tumors that can potentially be exploited to assess outcome after locoregional or targeted therapies.
- Although PET has been explored to characterize tumors before therapy and assess susceptibility to treatment, evidence from prospective randomized trials investigating the role of PET for response assessment after locoregional therapies are largely missing.

Disclosures: No conflicts of interests exist relevant to this article. Ms I. Schobert reports grants from the Biomedical Education Program (BMEP) outside the submitted work. Dr J. Chapiro reports grants from the German-Israeli Foundation for Scientific Research and Development, The Rolf W. Günther Foundation for Radiological Research, Boston Scientific, and Guerbet outside the submitted work. Dr L.J. Savic reports grants from Leopoldina Postdoctoral Fellowship outside the submitted work. Drs L.J. Savic and J. Chapiro report grants from National Institutes of Health (R01 CA206180) and the Society of Interventional Oncology outside the submitted work. All other authors have nothing to disclose.

[a] Department of Radiology and Biomedical Imaging, Yale University School of Medicine, 333 Cedar Street, New Haven, CT 06520, USA; [b] Institute of Radiology, Charité – Universitätsmedizin Berlin, Humboldt-Universität, Berlin Institute of Health, Augustenburger Platz 1, Berlin 13353, Germany
* Corresponding author. Department of Radiology and Biomedical Imaging, Yale University School of Medicine, 333 Cedar Street, New Haven, CT 06520.
E-mail address: lynn.savic@yale.edu

INTRODUCTION

Hepatocellular carcinoma (HCC) is the sixth most common cancer and the third leading cause of cancer-related deaths worldwide, with continuously increasing incidence rates.[1-4] Moreover, the liver represents a common metastatic site for a variety of malignancies including neuroendocrine tumors and colorectal carcinoma.[5] Because most patients with primary and secondary liver cancer present at advanced disease stages, they are no longer amenable to curative treatments such as surgical resection or radiofrequency ablation.[6]

In this setting, intra-arterial therapies (IAT) provide guideline-approved mainstay treatments with the potential for downstaging and bridging of patients to resection or transplantation.[7,8] Transarterial chemoembolization (TACE) is the most frequently performed IAT and constitutes the standard of care for intermediate-stage HCC with relatively preserved liver function (Barcelona Clinic of Liver Cancer stage [BCLC] B), and liver-dominant metastatic disease.[9,10] The rationale of these catheter-based therapies is premised on the fact that healthy liver tissue is predominantly supplied by the portal vein, whereas the feeding vessels of the hypervascular tumor primarily branch from the hepatic artery. Therefore, TACE enables deposition of high doses of chemotherapy to the tumor while sparing nontumoral liver tissue.[11] The tumoricidal activity of TACE combines ischemia-induced hypoxia and nutrient deprivation with drug-induced cytotoxic effects that lead to tumor necrosis.[12]

However, the efficacy of TACE remains limited because of local residual or recurrent disease that requires repeated treatments.[10] Specifically, individual variations of biological and physiologic characteristics of the tumor and its tumor microenvironment (TME) may alter the susceptibility and response to embolotherapies but are not yet well understood. Thus, functional and molecular imaging tools are needed for the quantitative pretreatment characterization of tumors and early assessment of treatment efficacy to inform personalized therapeutic decisions.

Response assessment after TACE is traditionally performed using morphologic imaging such as contrast-enhanced computed tomography (CT) or MR imaging. Established standard response criteria on conventional imaging are based on measurements of tumor size and enhancement and thus provide limited insight into biophysiologic tumor functions.

To overcome these limitations in the monitoring of TACE effects, functional imaging techniques can provide useful additional qualitative and quantitative information on cancer cell metabolism and interactions with the TME. The currently most important established functional imaging modalities for liver tumors are diffusion-weighted MR imaging, yielding information about tissue cellularity, perfusion imaging with contrast-enhanced ultrasonography, CT or MR imaging, studying tissue microcirculation, and liver-specific contrast-enhanced MR imaging for the imaging of hepatocellular function.[11,13,14] PET is a radiotracer-based approach and is commonly used to visualize metabolic processes in tumors, but with limited applications in liver cancer imaging.[15]

This article reviews the current role and possible future applications of PET for the diagnosis of primary and secondary liver malignancies and monitoring of tumor response to TACE.

TRANSARTERIAL CHEMOEMBOLIZATION

TACE is the most frequently used IAT and is recommended in the clinical guidelines for both primary and secondary liver tumors. Two main types of TACE can be distinguished: conventional TACE (cTACE) and drug-eluting beads (DEB)-TACE. During cTACE, chemotherapeutic drugs are brought into emulsion with microembolic radiopaque iodized oil (Lipiodol). The mixture is injected into the tumor-feeding arteries followed by embolic agents, such as microspheres or gelfoam. Owing to high treatment variability and the potential risk of systemic chemotherapy exposure after cTACE, DEB-TACE was developed to achieve drug release from administered microspheres in a prolonged and sustained manner with a favorable toxicity profile.[4,11,16]

Radiologic tumor response is commonly assessed 1 month after TACE.[17] Follow-up imaging includes pre-contrast as well as multiphasic contrast-enhanced CT or MR imaging to measure the reduction of tumor size and enhancing portions. As opposed to systemic chemotherapy, tumor shrinkage is not considered a prognostic marker for treatment efficacy after TACE and is particularly inappropriate in the case of transient swelling after embolotherapies.[8,18] Thus, the European Association for the Study of the Liver (EASL) and the European Organization for Research and Treatment of Cancer (EORTC) guidelines currently recommend tumor response assessment after TACE according to modified response evaluation criteria in solid tumors (mRECIST) criteria based on changes of the enhancing tumor diameter. In addition, evolution of enhancement-based response criteria has introduced two-dimensional EASL measuring the enhancing tumor area and three-dimensional quantitative EASL for the assessment of enhancing tumor volumes.[19,20]

However, besides devascularization and necrosis, TACE has complex early effects on the tumor, its metabolism, and the TME, which are not yet fully understood. Specifically, molecular heterogeneity of metabolic phenotypes between tumors and within the same tumor may have an impact on susceptibility to embolotherapies and may in turn be influenced by TACE-induced effects.[21] In this context, tumor recurrence after TACE can be explained by an adaptive tumor response to hypoxia and nutrient deprivation, which is reflected by the phenomenon of a latency period before recurrence becomes measurable on follow-up imaging.[22] Surviving cancer cells often present a more aggressive phenotype with increased expression levels of hypoxia-inducible factor (HIF)-1α and vascular endothelial growth factor (VEGF), as an adaptation mechanism to hypoxia.[23,24] In this setting, Flourine-18 flourodeoxyglucose (^{18}F-FDG) PET may help to understand individual tumor biology and monitor metabolic activity over the course of treatment to inform personalized diagnostic and therapeutic alorithms for locoregional therapies.

^{18}F-FLUORODEOXYGLUCOSE PET FOR RESPONSE ASSESSMENT AFTER TRANSARTERIAL CHEMOEMBOLIZATION

One of the hallmarks of cancer is the altered cancer metabolism that can be exploited for imaging purposes.[25] The characteristic metabolic shift of cancer cells to a hyperglycolytic phenotype implies the oxygen-independent reliance on glycolysis as the main axis of energy supply for cancer cells.[26] It has long been known as the "Warburg effect" or "aerobic glycolysis" and has recently gained new interest as a principal feature of tumorigenesis.[27] On a molecular level, the hyperglycolytic phenotype of tumor cells is defined by alterations of the expression levels of metabolic proteins. Upregulation of transmembrane glucose transporter (GLUT)-1 for increased glucose uptake has been demonstrated in many tumor types and emerges concomitant with malignant transformation.[28–31] FDG is a glucose analog that enters cancer cells via GLUT. The intracellular hexokinase II phosphorylates FDG into FDG-6-phosphate. This phosphorylated molecule cannot be further metabolized and accumulates intracellularly. As most malignant cells overexpress GLUT and hexokinase II, FDG accumulation in tumors can be exploited as the rationale for ^{18}F-FDG PET in the diagnosis, staging, and monitoring of many tumor types. At present, PET is mostly combined with CT

or MR imaging as hybrid imaging to increase precision and improve anatomic resolution. PET signal is usually quantified using standardized uptake value (SUV) and ratios of tumor to liver SUVs.[32,33] For tumor response assessment, standardized response criteria have been established, such as PET response criteria in solid tumors (PERCIST) and EORTC.[34]

However, ^{18}F-FDG PET is not commonly used and currently not included in clinical guidelines for the diagnostic workup of primary liver cancer. Specifically, PET/CT is not recommended by the National Comprehensive Network (NCCN) for the detection of HCC because of its limited sensitivity, although NCCN guidelines do acknowledge that higher HCC intralesional SUV is a marker of biological aggressiveness and may predict less optimal response to locoregional therapies.[35,36] Nevertheless, ^{18}F-FDG PET is included in NCCN algorithms of advanced solid cancers with a propensity for secondary spread to liver, such as colon, lung, and melanoma.[37]

Given the high metabolic activity of the liver, ^{18}F-FDG PET tumor imaging is limited by background signal from liver parenchyma, with consequent decreased sensitivity for detection of tumors with low avidity (ie, low-grade HCC) and low cellularity (ie, mucinous colon cancer metastasis or necrotic metastasis from any primary site). Clinical evidence on the utility of ^{18}F-FDG PET for tumor response assessment after locoregional therapies remains limited and largely controversial.

A large number of novel radiolabeled tracers is currently under investigation for the detection and monitoring of tumors and their TME. However, to date only few of these have been successfully translated into clinical routine. In particular, environmental factors such as altered pH and hypoxia are targets for molecular imaging in oncology.[38] Tumor hypoxia is considered to substantially contribute to tumor resistance to radiation as well conventional chemotherapy. Several trials have evaluated tumor hypoxia using different ^{18}F-labeled PET tracers that proved safe for clinical use in a phase 1 study of patients with lung cancer.[39] MR-based techniques include blood oxygen level-dependent (BOLD) MR imaging and ^{19}F-labeled MR imaging.[40,41]

Moreover, accelerated glycolysis also implies the synthesis of large amounts of lactate, which is transported via proton-coupled monocarboxylate transporters (MCT), leading to an acidification of the surrounding TME. Thus, the extracellular pH (pHe) simultaneously decreases as the level of aggressiveness of the tumor increases.[42] Novel MR imaging methods have been developed to image tumor acidosis including BIRDS (biosensor imaging of redundant deviation in shifts) and phosphorus-31 MR spectroscopy.[43–46] Preliminary studies demonstrated the ability for pHe mapping in vivo with both approaches to distinguish between invasive and less aggressive tumor growth.[47] Furthermore, a long-known MR contrast technique recently came into the scientific limelight again. This technique uses chemical exchange saturation transfer (CEST) for imaging of various compounds, for example, lactate (LATEST), which are indirectly visualized through water signal circumventing labeling or radioactive isotopes.[48]

In addition, several promising imaging methodologies are currently being developed to capture clinically relevant elements of the immune TME, such as zirconium-89-labeled nivolumab, which enables mapping of the biodistribution of PD-1-expressing tumor-infiltrating t-lymphocytes.[49]

Hepatocellular Carcinoma

^{18}F-FDG PET only plays a minor role in the diagnostic management of HCC. A meta-analysis of 22 studies with 1721 patients with HCC showed that ^{18}F-FDG PET/CT may be useful for predicting prognosis (ie, overall survival and disease-free survival, $P<.001$).[36] Another meta-analysis demonstrated the utility of ^{18}F-FDG PET/CT in ruling in extrahepatic metastases of HCC and ruling out recurrent HCC.[50] However, overall ^{18}F-FDG PET/CT has a low sensitivity for HCC detection.[51]

HCC typically exhibits a hyperglycolytic phenotype with increased glucose uptake facilitated by GLUT-1 overexpression.[52] As opposed to cancer cells, metabolic activity of hepatocytes comprises multiple pathways apart from glycolysis. Specifically, gluconeogenesis with high enzymatic activity of glucose-6-phosphatase can be found, which reduces intracellular accumulation of FDG in liver parenchyma.[53] However, glucose-6-phosphatase can also be found in malignant tumors at varying activity. Low-grade HCC in particular demonstrate glucose-6-phosphatase activities comparable with normal liver tissue, decreasing FDG uptake and, thus, diagnostic sensitivity of PET by 50% (**Table 1**).

On the other hand, large and high-grade HCC typically demonstrate increased ^{18}F-FDG uptake and thus can be detected using PET imaging with a high sensitivity of 83%.[54] As enhanced FDG uptake in HCC is associated with high serum levels of α-fetoprotein, p-glycoprotein expression, and increased VEGF levels, PET imaging can also be used to determine tumor differentiation and aggressiveness in a noninvasive manner.[55]

With regard to clinical evidence in the setting of locoregional therapies, a few studies exist that suggest an added prognostic value of PET imaging after TACE. Early studies dating back to 1994 already reported the heterogeneous FDG uptake behavior in tumors after TACE compared with normal liver parenchyma. Whereas viable tumor residuals demonstrated similar or increased uptake, decreased or absent uptake was associated with greater than 90% necrosis in explant histopathology.[56] Regarding quantitative analysis, an SUV reduction after TACE (SUV <3 or <3.5) compared with untreated tumors was shown to correlate with greater than 70%–80% tumor necrosis, indicating a positive clinical outcome.[57] In addition, decreased FDG uptake after TACE was an independent predictor of long-term survival after liver transplantation in patients with HCC.[58,59]

Among others, Song and colleagues evaluated ^{18}F-FDG PET/CT as a prognostic marker before TACE and for early response prediction after treatment. The investigators concluded that the uptake ratio SUV_{max} (tumor)/SUV_{mean} (liver) was a superior prognostic marker compared with tumor SUV alone. Specifically, cutoff ratios of less than 1.65 or 1.9, respectively, were determined to be predictive of tumor response after TACE. Nevertheless, with multiple factors influencing SUV, the application of universal absolute thresholds for tumor viability is not feasible.[60] Moreover, SUV ratio is strongly affected by the functional and metabolic state of the liver, making a baseline scan crucial to longitudinal evaluation of an individual patient's ratio over time.[61,62]

To improve the overall accuracy of PET for HCC, ^{18}F-FDG can be combined with carbon-11 (^{11}C)-acetate. ^{11}C-acetate enters cancer cells as a substrate for fatty acid synthesis, but its metabolization is poorly understood.[62,63] Several studies in HCC demonstrated an increase of sensitivity from 45% to 61% for ^{18}F-FDG PET alone to 73% to 83% for combined ^{18}F-FDG/^{11}C-acetate PET. However, this increased sensitivity was only confirmed for primary tumors and not for extrahepatic metastases of HCC. For small HCC (<2 cm), neither ^{18}F-FDG nor the combination with ^{11}C-acetate achieved reliable results, with low sensitivities of 27% and 32%, respectively. In terms of tumor differentiation, low-grade HCC showed higher uptake of ^{11}C-acetate in comparison with ^{18}F-FDG.[51,64]

Cholangiocarcinoma

There are only few trials investigating the value of PET for the diagnosis of cholangiocarcinoma (CC), with controversial findings. The detection accuracy of CC varies depending on the tumor

Table 1
Differential diagnosis of ^{18}F-FDG uptake

Differential Diagnosis	Examples	FDG Uptake (Compared with Liver)	Possibilities to Overcome Diagnostic Uncertainties
Inflammation	Lymphocytes, neutrophils, macrophages	↑	4-wk interval between TACE and PET
Infectious disease	Tuberculosis	↑	Review of clinical information
Benign tumors	Hemangioma	≈	Review contrast-enhanced MR imaging
	Focal nodular hyperplasia	≈ or slightly ↑	
Primary tumors	HCC	≈ (low-grade), ↑ (high grade)	Add ^{11}C-acetate to ^{18}F-FDG as a PET tracer
	ICC	≈ (infiltrative), ↑ (nodular)	Review contrast-enhanced MR imaging
Metastases	Colorectal, gastric, esophageal	↑ ≈ (mucinous mCRC)	Whole body PET scan + clinical information
	Neuroendocrine	≈ (low grade), ↑ (high grade)	Add somatostatin receptor imaging

Other Influential Factors			
Parameter	**Effect**		
Patient's age	Liver uptake	↑	Review clinical history and consider for image interpretation
Hepatic steatosis	Liver uptake	↑	
Tumor <1 cm	Sensitivity decreased		
Misregistration	Extrahepatic uptake or artifacts		
Incorrect attenuation correction in PET/CT			Review nonattenuation-corrected images as well

localization, with higher detection rates for intrahepatic CC (ICC) than for extrahepatic CC. Moreover, for intrahepatic tumors the sensitivity is high (85%) for nodular or mass-forming CC and low (18%) for infiltrating CC.[65] For the detection of regional lymph node metastases, MR imaging with MR cholangiopancreatography was clearly superior over ^{18}F-FDG PET. Distant metastases, however, were detected by PET at a high rate (about 100%) with an impact on the clinical management in up to 30% of patients, suggesting a beneficial role of ^{18}F-FDG PET for the staging of CC patients before therapy.[66]

Colorectal Cancer Metastases

In contrast to the management of HCC, the role of ^{18}F-FDG PET/CT or PET/MR imaging is more established in the detection, grading, and monitoring of colorectal cancer liver metastases (mCRC).[67] ^{18}F-FDG PET showed a mean sensitivity of 75% in detecting liver metastases.[68] However, although mCRC are generally FDG avid, mucinous subtypes, which account for 17% of mCRC, only show scarce uptake and are therefore difficult to diagnose.[69,70]

Ruers and colleagues investigated the impact of PET on the clinical outcome of mCRC patients. PET demonstrated a high sensitivity in identifying a noncurative setting and thus significantly reduced the number of liver resections that would be only beneficial with curative intent.[71] In addition, PET improved the detection of extrahepatic disease and thus changed the treatment plan in up to 38% of the patients.[72] Although the results of various studies confirm the higher sensitivity in detecting extrahepatic disease,[72–75] accuracy of detecting intrahepatic metastases using PET was similar to standard contrast-enhanced MR imaging and even inferior for the assessment of subcentimeter lesions. However, the overall accuracy of detecting intrahepatic and extrahepatic mCRC manifestations can possibly be improved by hybrid imaging with PET/MR imaging.[76]

Neuroendocrine Liver Metastases

Unlike in other malignancies, molecular imaging with PET is commonly applied for the diagnostic and therapeutic management of neuroendocrine tumors (NET). Radiolabeled somatostatin analogs represent the gold-standard imaging approach for most NET including liver metastases (NELM), but other tracers are under investigation. In this regard, PET/CT using gallium-68 (^{68}Ga)-conjugated somatostatin analog has a very high sensitivity (82%–100%) and specificity (67%–100%) in detecting (NELM).[68] ^{68}Ga-Dotatate PET/CT has recently been approved and incorporated into NCCN guidelines for NET.[37] Peptide receptor–targeted therapy with lutetium-177 (^{177}Lu) or yttrium-90 (^{90}Y)-labeled Dotatate is now used for NELM and is currently explored for combination with liver-targeted therapy. ^{68}Ga- and ^{177}Lu/^{90}Y-Dotatate represent a so-called theranostic pair, with the same agent used for diagnosis and therapy depending on the attached radionuclide.[77]

In addition, there are tumor-type–specific tracers that target molecular structures in NET subtypes such as glucagon-like peptide-1 receptor in insulinomas.[54] However, ^{18}F-FDG PET only proved beneficial for the monitoring of high-grade NELM because the overall sensitivity for NET detection was as low as 58%[78].

SUMMARY AND FUTURE DIRECTIONS: WHAT THE REFERRING PHYSICIAN NEEDS TO KNOW

To date, the efficacy of TACE has been hampered by a limited understanding of molecular changes induced in the tumor and its microenvironment over the course of treatment. Frequent tumor recurrence suggests that conventional tumor assessment on MR imaging or CT is insufficient to identify patients that are unlikely to respond. Although functional imaging techniques may generally help overcome these limitations, ^{18}F-FDG PET is not a guideline-approved tool for monitoring tumor response to embolotherapies in liver cancer. Nevertheless, as most liver tumors are hyperglycolytic, scientific evidence exists suggesting ^{18}F-FDG signal reduction as a functional biomarker for positive therapeutic outcome.[36] Thus, in addition to diagnostic implications for tumor detection, ^{18}F-FDG PET and combinations

with other dedicated radiotracers may be used to inform personalized treatment decisions and monitor tumor response to locoregional therapies such as TACE (**Box 1**).

Current clinical evidence only suggests limited added value of ^{18}F-FDG PET for the detection of extrahepatic metastases in HCC and the staging of CRLM.[79] However, the increasing understanding of tumor biology facilitated the identification of a variety of new molecular targets that can be exploited for both diagnostic and therapeutic purposes. In this regard, several prospective clinical trials in molecular imaging focus on the development of novel tracers with theranostic properties.[61,80] TACE may be combined with molecular targeted PET to monitor and target the biophysiologic tumor functions and create a favorable microenvironment for improved TACE efficacy.[81,82]

Several studies combined molecular targeted drugs with TACE, such as BRISK-TA, SPACE, ORIENTAL, and TACE-2.[83–85] As only a subset of patients responded to these newly introduced molecular therapies, new and reliable imaging techniques will be critical for identifying nonresponders early after therapy. PET and different radiotracers can be applied to complement morphologic imaging in this setting to achieve a

---

Box 1

Strengths and limitations of PET for the detection, grading, and monitoring of liver tumors after TACE

Strengths

- Functional information on metabolic activity of tumors
- Metabolic changes after treatment precede morphologic changes
- Combination of PET with CT or MR imaging increases sensitivity and specificity of imaging
- Combination of PET tracers (^{18}F-FDG + ^{11}C-acetate) increases sensitivity in HCC

Limitations

- Not guideline-approved for response assessment after TACE
- Sensitivity low for low-grade HCC, infiltrative ICC, mucinous mCRC
- Low spatial resolution (lesions <1 cm not detectable)
- ^{18}F-FDG is not tumor specific
- Lipiodol-induced attenuation correction artifacts of PET/CT
- High costs and duration

comprehensive characterization of the tumor and its microenvironment. This will help evaluate individual tumor susceptibility to a specific therapy and monitor early physiologic alterations in tumors before morphologic changes occur. These hybrid imaging methods may ultimately facilitate the successful application of locoregional therapies alone or in combination with new targeted agents in a more personalized fashion.

REFERENCES

1. Fong ZV, Tanabe KK. The clinical management of hepatocellular carcinoma in the United States, Europe, and Asia: a comprehensive and evidence-based comparison and review. Cancer 2014; 120(18):2824–38.
2. Lintoiu-Ursut B, Tulin A, Constantinoiu S. Recurrence after hepatic resection in colorectal cancer liver metastasis -Review article. J Med Life 2015;8(Spec Issue):12–4.
3. European Association for Study of Liver, European Organisation for Research and Treatment of Cancer. EASL-EORTC clinical practice guidelines: management of hepatocellular carcinoma. J Hepatol 2012; 56(4):908–43.
4. Lencioni R, de Baere T, Soulen MC, et al. Lipiodol transarterial chemoembolization for hepatocellular carcinoma: a systematic review of efficacy and safety data. Hepatology 2016;64(1):106–16.
5. Bray F, Ferlay J, Soerjomataram I, et al. Global cancer statistics 2018: GLOBOCAN estimates of incidence and mortality worldwide for 36 cancers in 185 countries. CA Cancer J Clin 2018;68(6): 394–424.
6. Wong MCS, Jiang JY, Goggins WB, et al. International incidence and mortality trends of liver cancer: a global profile. Sci Rep 2017;7:45846.
7. Wang DS, Louie JD, Sze DY. Intra-arterial therapies for metastatic colorectal cancer. Semin Interv Radiol 2013;30(1):12–20.
8. Bruix J, Sherman M. Management of hepatocellular carcinoma. Hepatology 2005;42(5):1208–36.
9. De Greef K, Rolfo C, Russo A, et al. Multidisciplinary management of patients with liver metastasis from colorectal cancer. World J Gastroenterol 2016; 22(32):7215–25.
10. Lewandowski RJ, Geschwind JF, Liapi E, et al. Transcatheter intraarterial therapies: rationale and overview. Radiology 2011;259(3):641–57.
11. Lencioni R, Petruzzi P, Crocetti L. Chemoembolization of hepatocellular carcinoma. Semin Interv Radiol 2013;30(1):3–11.
12. de Baere T, Arai Y, Lencioni R, et al. Treatment of liver tumors with lipiodol TACE: technical recommendations from experts opinion. Cardiovasc Intervent Radiol 2016;39(3):334–43.

13. Taouli B, Koh DM. Diffusion-weighted MR imaging of the liver. Radiology 2010;254(1):47–66.
14. Torizuka T, Tamaki N, Inokuma T, et al. In vivo assessment of glucose metabolism in hepatocellular carcinoma with FDG-PET. J Nucl Med 1995;36(10):1811–7.
15. Vilgrain V, Van Beers BE, Pastor CM. Insights into the diagnosis of hepatocellular carcinomas with hepatobiliary MRI. J Hepatol 2016;64(3):708–16.
16. Ronot M, Lambert S, Daire JL, et al. Can we justify not doing liver perfusion imaging in 2013? Diagn Interv Imaging 2013;94(12):1323–36.
17. Song JE, Kim DY. Conventional vs drug-eluting beads transarterial chemoembolization for hepatocellular carcinoma. World J Hepatol 2017;9(18):808–14.
18. Aghemo A. Update on HCC management and review of the new EASL guidelines. Gastroenterol Hepatol 2018;14(6):384–6.
19. Forner A, Ayuso C, Varela M, et al. Evaluation of tumor response after locoregional therapies in hepatocellular carcinoma: are response evaluation criteria in solid tumors reliable? Cancer 2009;115(3):616–23.
20. Kamel IR, Liapi E, Reyes DK, et al. Unresectable hepatocellular carcinoma: serial early vascular and cellular changes after transarterial chemoembolization as detected with MR imaging. Radiology 2009; 250(2):466–73.
21. Tacher V, Lin M, Duran R, et al. Comparison of existing response criteria in patients with hepatocellular carcinoma treated with transarterial chemoembolization using a 3D quantitative approach. Radiology 2016;278(1):275–84.
22. Roth GS, Decaens T. Liver immunotolerance and hepatocellular carcinoma: patho-physiological mechanisms and therapeutic perspectives. Eur J Cancer 2017;87:101–12.
23. Higuchi T, Kikuchi M, Okazaki M. Hepatocellular carcinoma after transcatheter hepatic arterial embolization. A histopathologic study of 84 resected cases. Cancer 1994;73(9):2259–67.
24. Liu K, Min XL, Peng J, et al. The changes of HIF-1alpha and VEGF expression after TACE in patients with hepatocellular carcinoma. J Clin Med Res 2016; 8(4):297–302.
25. Hanahan D, Weinberg RA. Hallmarks of cancer: the next generation. Cell 2011;144(5):646–74.
26. Gade TPF, Tucker E, Nakazawa MS, et al. Ischemia induces quiescence and autophagy dependence in hepatocellular carcinoma. Radiology 2017;283(3): 702–10.
27. Savic LJ, Chapiro J, Duwe G, et al. Targeting glucose metabolism in cancer: new class of agents for loco-regional and systemic therapy of liver cancer and beyond? Hepat Oncol 2016;3(1):19–28.
28. Warburg O, Gawehn K, Geissler AW. The transformation of embryonal metabolism in cancer metabolism. Z Naturforsch B 1960;15B:378–9 [in German].

29. Lunt SY, Vander Heiden MG. Aerobic glycolysis: meeting the metabolic requirements of cell proliferation. Annu Rev Cell Dev Biol 2011;27:441–64.

30. Warburg O, Wind F, Negelein E. The metabolism of tumors in the body. J Gen Physiol 1927;8(6):519–30.

31. Warburg O. On the origin of cancer cells. Science 1956;123(3191):309–14.

32. Martinez GV, Zhang X, García-Martín ML, et al. Imaging the extracellular pH of tumors by MRI after injection of a single cocktail of T1 and T2 contrast agents. NMR Biomed 2011;24(10):1380–91.

33. Beiderwellen K, Geraldo L, Ruhlmann V, et al. Accuracy of [^{18}F]FDG PET/MRI for the detection of liver metastases. PLoS One 2015;10(9):e0137285.

34. Beiderwellen K, Gomez B, Buchbender C, et al. Depiction and characterization of liver lesions in whole body [(1)(8)F]-FDG PET/MRI. Eur J Radiol 2013;82(11):e669–75.

35. Benson AB, D'Angelica MI, Abbott DE, et al. Guidelines insights: hepatobiliary cancers, version 2.2019. J Natl Compr Canc Netw 2019;17(4):302–10.

36. Sun DW, An L, Wei F, et al. Prognostic significance of parameters from pretreatment (18)F-FDG PET in hepatocellular carcinoma: a meta-analysis. Abdom Radiol (NY) 2016;41(1):33–41.

37. Shah MH, Goldner WS, Halfdanarson TR, et al. NCCN guidelines insights: neuroendocrine and Adrenal tumors, version 2.2018. J Natl Compr Canc Netw 2018;16(6):693–702.

38. Pinker K, Riedl C, Weber WA. Evaluating tumor response with FDG PET: updates on PERCIST, comparison with EORTC criteria and clues to future developments. Eur J Nucl Med Mol Imaging 2017; 44(Suppl 1):55–66.

39. Buck MD, Sowell RT, Kaech SM, et al. Metabolic instruction of immunity. Cell 2017;169(4):570–86.

40. Peeters SG, Zegers CM, Lieuwes NG, et al. A comparative study of the hypoxia PET tracers [^{18}F]HX4, [^{18}F]FAZA, and [^{18}F]FMISO in a preclinical tumor model. Int J Radiat Oncol Biol Phys 2015; 91(2):351–9.

41. Savi A, Incerti E, Fallanca F, et al. First evaluation of PET-based human biodistribution and dosimetry of ^{18}F-FAZA, a tracer for imaging tumor hypoxia. J Nucl Med 2017;58(8):1224–9.

42. Lopci E, Grassi I, Chiti A, et al. PET radiopharmaceuticals for imaging of tumor hypoxia: a review of the evidence. Am J Nucl Med Mol Imaging 2014;4(4): 365–84.

43. Végran F, Boidot R, Michiels C, et al. Lactate influx through the endothelial cell monocarboxylate transporter MCT1 supports an NF-κB/IL-8 pathway that drives tumor angiogenesis. Cancer Res 2011; 71(7):2550–60.

44. Pértega-Gomes N, Vizcaíno JR, Miranda-Gonçalves V, et al. Monocarboxylate transporter 4 (MCT4) and CD147 overexpression is associated with poor prognosis in prostate cancer. BMC Cancer 2011;11:312.

45. Feron O. Pyruvate into lactate and back: from the Warburg effect to symbiotic energy fuel exchange in cancer cells. Radiother Oncol 2009;92(3):329–33.

46. Pinheiro C, Longatto-Filho A, Azevedo-Silva J, et al. Role of monocarboxylate transporters in human cancers: state of the art. J Bionerg Biomembr 2012; 44(1):127–39. Springer Science+Business Media.

47. Gillies RJ, Raghunand N, Karczmar GS, et al. MRI of the tumor microenvironment. J Magn Reson Imaging 2002;16(4):430–50.

48. Coman D, Huang Y, Rao JU, et al. Imaging the intratumoral-peritumoral extracellular pH gradient of gliomas. NMR Biomed 2016;29(3):309–19.

49. DeBrosse C, Nanga RP, Bagga P, et al. Lactate chemical exchange saturation transfer (LATEST) imaging in vivo A biomarker for LDH activity. Sci Rep 2016;6:19517.

50. Lin CY, Chen JH, Liang JA, et al. ^{18}F-FDG PET or PET/CT for detecting extrahepatic metastases or recurrent hepatocellular carcinoma: a systematic review and meta-analysis. Eur J Radiol 2012;81(9): 2417–22.

51. Park JW, Kim JH, Kim SK, et al. A prospective evaluation of ^{18}F-FDG and ^{11}C-acetate PET/CT for detection of primary and metastatic hepatocellular carcinoma. J Nucl Med 2008;49(12):1912–21.

52. England CG, Jiang D, Ehlerding EB, et al. (89)Zr-labeled nivolumab for imaging of T-cell infiltration in a humanized murine model of lung cancer. Eur J Nucl Med Mol Imaging 2018;45(1):110–20.

53. Amann T, Maegdefrau U, Hartmann A, et al. GLUT1 expression is increased in hepatocellular carcinoma and promotes tumorigenesis. Am J Pathol 2009; 174(4):1544–52.

54. Ronot M, Clift AK, Vilgrain V, et al. Functional imaging in liver tumours. J Hepatol 2016;65(5):1017–30.

55. Kornberg A, Schernhammer M, Friess H. (18)F-FDG-PET for assessing biological viability and prognosis in liver transplant patients with hepatocellular carcinoma. J Clin Transl Hepatol 2017;5(3):224–34.

56. Seo S, Hatano E, Higashi T, et al. Fluorine-18 fluorodeoxyglucose positron emission tomography predicts tumor differentiation, P-glycoprotein expression, and outcome after resection in hepatocellular carcinoma. Clin Cancer Res 2007;13(2 Pt 1):427–33.

57. Torizuka T, Tamaki N, Inokuma T, et al. Value of fluorine-18-FDG-PET to monitor hepatocellular carcinoma after interventional therapy. J Nucl Med 1994; 35(12):1965–9.

58. Cascales Campos P, Ramirez P, Gonzalez R, et al. Value of 18-FDG-positron emission tomography/computed tomography before and after transarterial chemoembolization in patients with hepatocellular carcinoma undergoing liver transplantation: initial results. Transplant Proc 2011;43(6):2213–5.

59. Cascales-Campos PA, Ramirez P, Lopez V, et al. Prognostic value of 18-fluorodeoxyglucose-positron emission tomography after transarterial chemoembolization in patients with hepatocellular carcinoma undergoing orthotopic liver transplantation. Transplant Proc 2015;47(8):2374–6.

60. Kornberg A, Witt U, Matevossian E, et al. Extended postinterventional tumor necrosis-implication for outcome in liver transplant patients with advanced HCC. PLoS One 2013;8(1):e53960.

61. Song MJ, Bae SH, Lee SW, et al. ^{18}F-fluorodeoxyglucose PET/CT predicts tumour progression after transarterial chemoembolization in hepatocellular carcinoma. Eur J Nucl Med Mol Imaging 2013;40(6):865–73.

62. Song MJ, Bae SH, Yoo Ie R, et al. Predictive value of (1)(8)F-fluorodeoxyglucose PET/CT for transarterial chemolipiodolization of hepatocellular carcinoma. World J Gastroenterol 2012;18(25):3215–22.

63. Petrides AS, DeFronzo RA. Glucose and insulin metabolism in cirrhosis. J Hepatol 1989;8(1):107–14.

64. Li S, Peck-Radosavljevic M, Ubl P, et al. The value of [(11)C]-acetate PET and [(18)F]-FDG PET in hepatocellular carcinoma before and after treatment with transarterial chemoembolization and bevacizumab. Eur J Nucl Med Mol Imaging 2017;44(10):1732–41.

65. Ho CL, Yu SC, Yeung DW. ^{11}C-acetate PET imaging in hepatocellular carcinoma and other liver masses. J Nucl Med 2003;44(2):213–21.

66. Anderson CD, Rice MH, Pinson CW, et al. Fluorodeoxyglucose PET imaging in the evaluation of gallbladder carcinoma and cholangiocarcinoma. J Gastrointest Surg 2004;8(1):90–7.

67. Petrowsky H, Wildbrett P, Husarik DB, et al. Impact of integrated positron emission tomography and computed tomography on staging and management of gallbladder cancer and cholangiocarcinoma. J Hepatol 2006;45(1):43–50.

68. Brendle C, Schwenzer NF, Rempp H, et al. Assessment of metastatic colorectal cancer with hybrid imaging: comparison of reading performance using different combinations of anatomical and functional imaging techniques in PET/MRI and PET/CT in a short case series. Eur J Nucl Med Mol Imaging 2016;43(1):123–32.

69. Kinkel K, Lu Y, Both M, et al. Detection of hepatic metastases from cancers of the gastrointestinal tract by using noninvasive imaging methods (US, CT, MR imaging, PET): a meta-analysis. Radiology 2002;224(3):748–56.

70. Bipat S, van Leeuwen MS, Comans EF, et al. Colorectal liver metastases: CT, MR imaging, and PET for diagnosis–meta-analysis. Radiology 2005;237(1):123–31.

71. Grassetto G, Capirci C, Marzola MC, et al. Colorectal cancer: prognostic role of ^{18}F-FDG-PET/CT. Abdom Imaging 2012;37(4):575–9.

72. Ruers TJ, Wiering B, van der Sijp JR, et al. Improved selection of patients for hepatic surgery of colorectal liver metastases with (18)F-FDG PET: a randomized study. J Nucl Med 2009;50(7):1036–41.

73. Yang YY, Fleshman JW, Strasberg SM. Detection and management of extrahepatic colorectal cancer in patients with resectable liver metastases. J Gastrointest Surg 2007;11(7):929–44.

74. Huebner RH, Park KC, Shepherd JE, et al. A meta-analysis of the literature for whole-body FDG PET detection of recurrent colorectal cancer. J Nucl Med 2000;41(7):1177–89.

75. Wiering B, Krabbe PF, Jager GJ, et al. The impact of fluor-18-deoxyglucose-positron emission tomography in the management of colorectal liver metastases. Cancer 2005;104(12):2658–70.

76. Sahani DV, Kalva SP, Fischman AJ, et al. Detection of liver metastases from adenocarcinoma of the colon and pancreas: comparison of mangafodipir trisodium-enhanced liver MRI and whole-body FDG PET. AJR Am J Roentgenol 2005;185(1):239–46.

77. Werner RA, Bluemel C, Allen-Auerbach MS, et al. [68]Gallium- and [90]Yttrium-/[177]Lutetium: "theranostic twins" for diagnosis and treatment of NETs. Ann Nucl Med 2015;29(1):1–7.

78. Kiesewetter DO, Gao H, Ma Y, et al. ^{18}F-radiolabeled analogs of exendin-4 for PET imaging of GLP-1 in insulinoma. Eur J Nucl Med Mol Imaging 2012;39(3):463–73.

79. Armbruster M, Zech CJ, Sourbron S, et al. Diagnostic accuracy of dynamic gadoxetic-acid-enhanced MRI and PET/CT compared in patients with liver metastases from neuroendocrine neoplasms. J Magn Reson Imaging 2014;40(2):457–66.

80. Song HJ, Cheng JY, Hu SL, et al. Value of ^{18}F-FDG PET/CT in detecting viable tumour and predicting prognosis of hepatocellular carcinoma after TACE. Clin Radiol 2015;70(2):128–37.

81. Wang CH, Wey KC, Mo LR, et al. Current trends and recent advances in diagnosis, therapy, and prevention of hepatocellular carcinoma. Asian Pac J Cancer Prev 2015;16(9):3595–604.

82. Minguez B, Tovar V, Chiang D, et al. Pathogenesis of hepatocellular carcinoma and molecular therapies. Curr Opin Gastroenterol 2009;25(3):186–94.

83. Kallini JR, Miller FH, Gabr A, et al. Hepatic imaging following intra-arterial embolotherapy. Abdom Radiol (NY) 2016;41(4):600–16.

84. Samim M, El-Haddad GE, Molenaar IQ, et al. [18F] Fluorodeoxyglucose PET for interventional oncology in liver malignancy. PET Clin 2014;9(4):469–95, vi.

85. Wang G, Liu Y, Zhou SF, et al. Sorafenib combined with transarterial chemoembolization in patients with hepatocellular carcinoma: a meta-analysis and systematic review. Hepatol Int 2016;10(3):501–10.

The Unique Role of Fluorodeoxyglucose-PET in Radioembolization

Remco Bastiaannet, Msc[a,b], Martin A. Lodge, MS, PhD[b],
Hugo W.A.M. de Jong, PhD[a], Marnix G.E.H. Lam, MD, PhD[a,*]

KEYWORDS

- Radioembolization • Metabolic response assessment • Dose–response • FDG-PET

KEY POINTS

- Pretreatment metabolic metrics can predict progression-free survival and overall survival.
- Metabolic response metrics predict treatment response or survival earlier and are more accurate than morphologic measures (eg, response evaluation criteria in solid tumors [RECIST]).
- Fluorodeoxyglucose (FDG)-avidity may serve as a clinically relevant method for treatment target volume definition.
- Metabolic response correlates well with estimates of absorbed tumor dose derived from yttrium-90 PET/computed tomography (^{90}Y PET/CT).
- There is currently little convergence toward standardization or consensus regarding the optimal metabolic metric. The relevant metric might be tumor type-specific.

INTRODUCTION

Radioembolization is becoming an established treatment of unresectable, chemorefractory, primary and secondary liver tumors. It consists of the intraarterial infusion of millions of microspheres loaded with yttrium-90 (^{90}Y) into the hepatic vasculature. Due to the dual blood supply of the liver, the microspheres mostly accumulate in the tumorous tissue, resulting in a local radiation dose to the tumor while minimizing the dose to healthy liver tissue. The therapy is preceded by a safety procedure in which extrahepatic deposition and the amount of lung shunting is established.

The efficacy of adding radioembolization to first-line treatments for metastatic colorectal carcinoma (mCRC) was studied in the randomized controlled trials SIRFLOX,[1] FOXFIRE,[2] and FOXFIRE-Global. These trials did not show a significant improvement in either progression-free survival (PFS)[3] or overall survival (OS).[4] The treatment of advanced hepatocellular carcinoma (HCC) with SIR-spheres versus sorafenib was investigated in the SARAH and SIRveNIB phase III studies, which also failed to show an improvement in OS or PFS.[5,6]

It has been suggested that the reasons that these trials did not meet their primary endpoints were due to issues related to patient selection and an insufficiently personalized and suboptimal dosimetry.[7–9] Better survival may be achieved with improved patient selection and dosimetry. Furthermore, improved response monitoring can guide these

Disclosure: This work has been partially supported by the ENEN + project that has received funding from the Euratom research and training work programme #755576 (R. Bastiaannet) and Siemens Medical Solutions (H.W.A.M. de Jong). This project has received funding from the European Research Council (ERC) under the European Union's Horizon 2020 research and innovation program (grant no [646734]) (H.W.A.M. de Jong).

[a] Department of Radiology and Nuclear Medicine, University Medical Center, Huispost E01.132, Postbus 85500, Utrecht 3508 GA, Netherlands; [b] The Russell H. Morgan Department of Radiology and Radiological Science, Johns Hopkins University School of Medicine, 601 N. Caroline St., Baltimore, MD 21287, USA
* Corresponding author.
E-mail address: M.Lam@umcutrecht.nl

PET Clin 14 (2019) 447–457
https://doi.org/10.1016/j.cpet.2019.06.002
1556-8598/19/© 2019 Elsevier Inc. All rights reserved.

advancements in clinical studies, as well as improve the management of individual patients.[10]

Radioembolization is a locoregional treatment of hepatic tumors only. Therefore, a limited prognosis and extensive extrahepatic disease (EHD) burden are contraindications for treatment with radioembolization.[11,12] Accurate information on patient-specific tumor biology and the extent of EHD are crucial for patient selection. The capability of imaging metabolic processes by fluorodeoxyglucose (FDG)-PET might contribute to a more informed patient selection.

For an improved dosimetry, it is crucial to be able to determine tumor masses and to predict the subsequent activities administered to these masses.[7] The process of defining lesions and applying this to dose maps is greatly aided by the functional information provided by FDG-PET. Furthermore, improved accuracy and earlier response monitoring may help in posttreatment disease management. Metabolic imaging might be able to provide this.

These applications of FDG-PET depend on the target tumors being sufficiently FDG-avid. This is mainly the case for mCRC, less for HCC and intrahepatic cholangiocellular carcinoma (ICC), and limited for neuroendocrine tumors. This article focuses on the first 3 tumor types and reviews the unique role that FDG-PET may have in radioembolization for (1) improved patient selection and prognosis, (2) more personalized treatment planning, and (3) more accurate treatment response assessment. These 3 areas constitute key aspects of the treatment with radioembolization.

PATIENT SELECTION

It is currently recommended that EHD is established using triple-phasic contrast-enhanced computed tomography (CT) and/or gadolinium-enhanced MR imaging.[11] However, it has been shown that the addition of FDG-PET can lead to a higher sensitivity for EHD detection.

In a meta-analysis of 12 studies on the impact of PET on therapeutic management of mCRC, Maffione, and colleagues[13] found that PET findings changed disease management in 24% of subjects. This was commonly due to a switch from intended curative surgery to palliative treatment because previously unknown EHD burden was found. However, EHD detection rates varied from 0% to 68% of the included subjects in these studies. The investigators suggested that this might be explained by differences in study design and possibly selection bias of the included subjects.

Relative to contrast-enhanced CT and MR imaging, the use of FDG-PET/CT led to a change in mCRC disease management in 17% of the cases, due to a higher detection rate of EHD, in a study by Kong and colleagues.[14] However, the investigators recommended the use of manganese dipyridoxyl diphosphate liver MR imaging for intrahepatic disease owing to its superior sensitivity for small liver metastases.

Similar studies were performed more specifically in the context of radioembolization. Rosenbaum and colleagues[15] compared EHD detection between CT and FDG-PET, and its influence on decisions to treat mCRC with radioembolization. They found that FDG-PET found significantly more cases of EHD than CT alone, which resulted in a change in disease management in 7 out of 42 (17%) subjects.

In a study by Denecke and colleagues,[16] a sequential diagnostic algorithm to assess suitability for radioembolization was tested in 22 mCRC subjects. These subjects first underwent contrast-enhanced CT, which lead to the exclusion of 18% of the subjects owing to contraindications. Next, in the resulting group, a further 5 subjects (23% of total) were excluded after additional contraindications were found using FDG-PET.

In a study of 135 subjects with multifocal liver metastases, sensitivity for the detection of EHD by FDG-PET/CT was compared with whole-body MR imaging.[17] FDG-PET/CT and whole-body MR imaging were consecutively used to assess subject suitability for radioembolization. Of the exclusions, 91% were due to a significant EHD. Both FDG-PET/CT and MR imaging showed a high sensitivity and specificity, with FDG-PET/CT showing a trend to higher diagnostic accuracy.

There are some, albeit fewer, studies on the use of FDG-PET in HCC. For instance, in a study in 87 HCC subjects by Yoon and colleagues,[18] FDG-PET was more sensitive and detected 10 more cases of EHD than CT or MR imaging in the same group of subjects. As a consequence, 4 cases were upstaged because of additional findings.

In conclusion, these studies show that FDG-PET is more sensitive to the presence of EHD and, in the case of mCRC, leads to changes in disease management in around 20% of patients compared with anatomic imaging alone.

Pretreatment Metabolism as a Prognostic Factor

Anatomic metrics, such as the response evaluation criteria in solid tumors (RECIST), have been the recommended indicators for the assessment of treatment response after radioembolization.[11] However, the use of tumor size alone is problematic in many cases, such as in the presence of substantial necrosis. In these cases, tumor morphology may not accurately reflect tumor viability. Conversely, FDG uptake is proportional to the number of viable tumor cells present in a volume of tissue.[19] In addition, when measured with FDG-PET, the standardized uptake value (SUV) is a physiologically relevant measure of cell metabolism.[20,21] As such, FDG uptake may reflect the nature of the tumor biology, and thus disease progression, more accurately.

A minimal life expectancy of 6 months is generally recommended before treatment with radioembolization.[11] Pretreatment prognostic information can potentially refine patient selection before radioembolization. There are several studies in the literature that show such a link between pretreatment liver tumor metabolism and survival after treatment with radioembolization.

In a prospective trial, in which 90 mCRC subjects underwent an FDG-PET scan before hepatectomy, Riedl and colleagues[22] were able to correlate maximal SUV (SUV_{max}) to the expression of histologic markers for cell proliferation, glucose transport, and cell cycle control. Furthermore, survival was significantly longer for subjects with a low SUV_{max}.

In the case of liver metastasized breast cancer, Haug and colleagues[23] found that a high pretreatment SUV_{max} of the liver tumors was significantly associated with a shorter survival (21 vs 52 weeks). Similar findings were published for ICC by Soydal and colleagues.[24] Baseline FDG avidity, the dimensions of the largest lesion, and pretreatment tumor load were predictive of OS. For uveal melanoma, it was found that baseline total lesion glycolysis (TLG), not SUV_{max}, was predictive of OS and PFS.[25] In addition, for metastatic melanoma, it was neither SUV_{max} nor TLG but rather the fraction of the liver volume that was metabolically active that was a prognostic marker of survival.[26]

A similar link was shown for HCC, in which FDG-avidity at baseline was a significant predictor of OS.[27] An SUV_{max} higher than 3 was shown to be associated with decreased tumor control and a decreased PFS in HCC by Abuodeh and colleagues.[28] Interestingly, Jreige and colleagues[29] found that, in HCC subjects, pretreatment SUV_{max} and the tumor-to-liver uptake ratio were significant negative prognostic markers for both PFS and OS but morphologic metrics such as size and number of hepatic tumors were not. This is in line with a large meta-analysis of 1721 HCC subjects who received standard of care treatment reaching the same conclusion.[30]

Taken together, these studies indicate that pretreatment hepatic tumor metabolism is a significant predictor of OS and/or PFS for several tumor types. Furthermore, FDG metabolism was linked to the expression of GLUT1, Ki67, and p53, which are markers associated with tumor aggressiveness.[22,31] However, there seems to be no current consensus on which exact metabolic metric (eg, TLG or SUV_{max}) should be used.

DETERMINING THE TARGET VOLUME

As previously described, FDG-avidity is linked to tumor aggressiveness and viability, and to patient survival. The metabolic tumor volume (MTV) is defined as all parts of the lesion that are comparatively FDG-avid. This provides a convenient definition of target volume for treatment, consisting of the most clinically relevant parts of the tumor.[32,33] These target volumes may be used for treatment planning using the partition model,[34] or for tumor absorbed dose–response studies.[35] A typical example of the heterogeneity of tumor FDG uptake is shown in **Fig. 1**A. This heterogeneity would be largely ignored when determining the target volume based on anatomic imaging only. An example

A

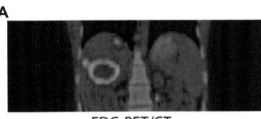

FDG-PET/CT

B

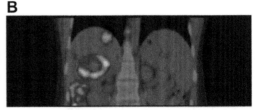

Posttreatment ^{90}Y PET/CT

Fig. 1. Good spatial correspondence between tumor FDG-uptake and microsphere deposition. The main target lesion in (A) exhibits the typical characteristics of a heterogeneous tumor with a nonviable, necrotic core. This heterogeneity will result in discrepancies between anatomically (including necrosis) and metabolically defined target volumes. Coregistration of the CTs of (A) and (B) allows for the application of this metabolic mask to the posttreatment scan. The microspheres in (B) accumulated mostly in the viable parts of the tumor, depositing most of their dose in the viable regions. The use of anatomically or metabolically defined masks is likely to result in very different dose estimates for this patient.

in which this difference would be pronounced is given in **Fig. 1**.

There are many ways to define the MTV.[36] The exact segmentation method used is commonly determined by practical reasons, such as clinical convenience, appropriate analysis software, or adherence to specific guidelines. The exact choice of delineation strategy, however, has an effect on the accuracy of the extracted quantity,[37] its reproducibility in the clinic,[38] and its value for therapy planning and monitoring. Especially for the latter, the combination of tumor type and treatment modality might dictate the appropriate method.[7,39] Most of the current studies either rely on manual segmentation or threshold-based segmentations.

The relative differences in delineation methods are illustrated in **Fig. 2**.

Manual segmentation is perhaps the most intuitive and seemingly robust way to segment a PET or anatomic scan. This method makes full use of the radiologist's experience, context awareness, and high-level knowledge of artifacts (eg, noise, patient motion, partial volume effects). However, it is very time-consuming and is prone to high interoperator and intraoperator variability.[40,41] In part, this variability can be attributed to the ambiguity caused by partial volume effects.[36,40] A possible solution is to statistically weigh segmentations from multiple readers to arrive at an optimal segmentation, but this requires a large number of readers for each scan, reducing practicality.[42]

Threshold-based methods try to extract the MTV (high FDG uptake) from the background (low FDG uptake) by setting an SUV threshold value. This value may simply be an absolute value (eg, SUV >2.5). This was shown to carry great prognostic value in lung cancer, as shown in a meta-analysis by Im and colleagues.[43] However,

the actual volumes of tumors with a low uptake are likely to be underestimated with this method owing to the partial volume effect.[44]

Thresholds are more commonly chosen relative to either SUV_{max}[45] or to the uptake in another region within the body (eg, blood pool[35] or liver uptake[46]). For example, in a study by van den Hoven and colleagues,[35] a subject-relative SUV threshold (2 times the mean SUV normalized for lean body mass, measured in the aortic blood) was used, resulting in a semiautomatic, objective, and reproducible segmentation of the MTV. By subsequently using registration of the corresponding CTs, these masks can be transferred to both pretreatment and posttreatment scans.

TREATMENT RESPONSE ASSESSMENT

Besides carrying important prognostic information, FDG-PET can also be used to assess and quantify treatment response. Again, by reflecting changes in regional tumor metabolism, instead of anatomic morphology, FDG-PET is able to make more accurate predictions of treatment outcome and survival. More accurate response characterization is beneficial for informed decisions surrounding the treatment of an individual patient but can also act as a more accurate surrogate endpoint in clinical trials, increasing statistical power.[10,47,48] This notion is part of a much broader discussion that extends well beyond radioembolization. However, this article summarizes the relevant findings and their implications in the context of radioembolization.

Accuracy of Metabolic Response Assessment

Earlier studies primarily used visual assessment and/or consensus reading to categorize treatment

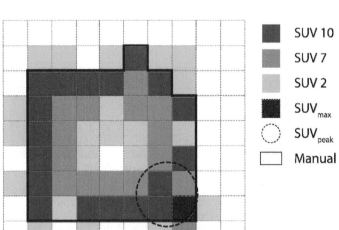

SUV 10
SUV 7
SUV 2
SUV_{max}
SUV_{peak}
Manual

Fig. 2. The potential differences and increasing degree of subjectivity of selecting SUV_{max}, peak SUV (SUV_{peak}), or manual segmentation to extract metabolic information. SUV_{peak} is commonly defined as the mean SUV within a 1 mL sphere positioned so as to have its maximum value. Of particular interest is that a great deal of experience and subjectivity is involved in the manual segmentation of tumors on PET.

response and to establish the feasibility of measuring changes in tumor metabolism after radioembolization.[49,50] Around the same time, comparing changes in FDG uptake with anatomic changes in a small cohort of 5 subjects revealed that there was a significant metabolic response at 1-month follow-up that did not correlate with the wide range of posttreatment changes observed on CT, such as both increases and decreases in tissue attenuation and lesion size, as well as the development of necrotic features.[51] This finding was replicated in many other studies for different tumor types.

Miller and colleagues[52] included subjects with unresectable liver metastases from various primary tumors in a comprehensive study comparing RECIST, WHO, necrosis-criteria, and PET-based response measures. In this study, the subjects underwent CT and PET scans immediately before treatment and at approximately 30 days after treatment, and in 60-day to 90-day intervals afterward. They found that the inclusion of necrosis or the combined RECIST plus necrosis criteria allowed for significantly earlier detection of response (around 1 month posttreatment) relative to WHO and RECIST (around 2–3 months posttreatment). This suggests that there is a significant impact of necrosis (and related physiology) on purely anatomic metrics, decreasing their sensitivity of early treatment response detection. Bienert and colleagues[51] provided a similar explanation but noted the potential difficulty of measuring necrotic features in more hypovascular tumors such as mCRC, emphasizing the utility of functional imaging for treatment response assessment.

In mCRC, some studies found that SUV_{max}, and not RECIST, predicted PFS,[53,54] whereas others found TLG and MTV to predict survival.[55–57] Interestingly, Jongen and colleagues[57] found a significant association of TLG with OS at 1-month and 3-month follow-up but for RECIST only at 3-month follow-up. Most of these studies cited the level of subjectivity for tumor measurement on CT, the limited effect of the treatment on tumor size, and the hypovascularity of mCRC as underlying causes for the superior accuracy of metabolic metrics for the prediction of survival. An example of an mCRC case, in which the metabolic response preceded the anatomic response, is given in **Fig. 3**.

Two studies that included ICC subjects exclusively, found that, at 3-month follow-up, changes in tumor metabolism did but anatomic metrics did not predict survival.[58,59] Similarly, Michl and colleagues[60] found that both peak SUV (SUV_{peak}) and changes in TLG predicted OS, PFS, and time to progression for subjects with metastatic pancreatic cancer.

Sabet and colleagues[27] showed that in HCC patients, changes in the ratio of SUV_{max} to background SUV ($SUV_{background}$) was a predictor of OS at 1-month follow-up.

Although it might be possible that the metabolic response is transient, these studies showed that changes in functional metrics following treatment could predict survival both more accurately and, in many cases, earlier (at 1-month follow-up rather than at 3-month follow-up) than anatomic metrics.[51,52,57] Early and reliable response assessment may aid decisions regarding subsequent treatments.

Correlating Absorbed Dose with Metabolic Response and Survival

With the advent of PET/CT scanners and reconstruction algorithms capable of ^{90}Y imaging, it became possible to directly investigate the relationship between tumor absorbed dose and response.[61–64] In these studies, radioembolization was generally approached as an internal radiotherapy modality. The aim of these studies was to investigate the potential utility of tumor absorbed dose optimization and local response prediction. An example is given in **Fig. 1**, in which FDG tumor uptake acted as a method for tumor definition that could serve as a mask for tumor absorbed dose calculations. **Table 1** is an overview of the most relevant studies that have used FDG PET/CT to quantify treatment response and have correlated this to tumor absorbed dose.

Flamen and colleagues[46] defined metabolic response as a TLG reduction that was larger than 50%. Metabolic response was associated with an estimated median absorbed dose of 46 Gy, whereas nonresponding tumors absorbed a median 20 Gy. This was corroborated by Willowson and colleagues,[65] who found an average absorbed dose of approximately 50 Gy to yield a significant response (>50% TLG reduction). Furthermore, a reduction in TLG greater than 65% was associated with improved OS. van den Hoven and colleagues[35] also found that tumor absorbed dose and TLG reduction correlated well (and depended on baseline TLG), and that a TLG reduction greater than 50% was associated with a prolonged OS. Levillain and colleagues[66] further confirmed this absorbed dose to TLG reduction correlation.

As previously described, anatomic metrics are generally less sensitive to measure response in mCRC. As a consequence, the studies in **Table 1** used metabolic response to assess treatment response in this tumor type, which resulted in significant relationships between the absorbed dose to the tumor and metabolic response.

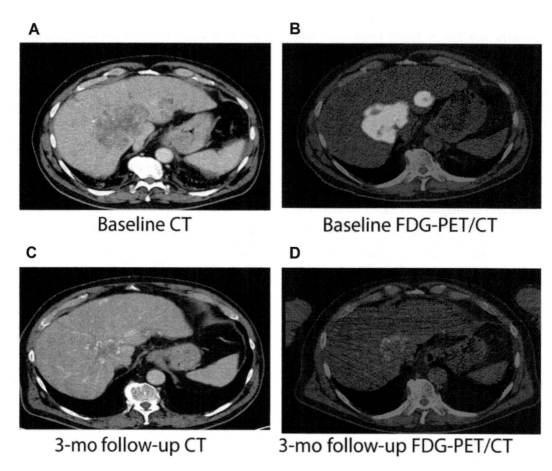

A

Baseline CT

B

Baseline FDG-PET/CT

C

3-mo follow-up CT

D

3-mo follow-up FDG-PET/CT

Fig. 3. Patient presented with substantial mCRC burden as evident on CT (*A*), which was metabolically active (*B*). Anatomic imaging at 3-month follow-up showed clear evidence of noncomplete response (*C*). Conversely, FDG-PET/CT showed a complete metabolic response at follow-up (*D*). The metabolic response precedes the anatomic response in this patient.

Unfortunately, every study in this table uses resin microspheres. It may be possible that glass microspheres have a different impact on tumor metabolism. An overview of recent absorbed dose response studies, including other tumor types and response metrics, is detailed elsewhere.[7]

THE OPTIMAL METABOLIC PARAMETER

The previously mentioned studies frequently used SUV_{max} as a quantitative metric to predict treatment outcome and survival. SUV_{max} is an attractive choice because it is both easily calculated on clinical workstations and is thought to have a direct relationship to the underlying tumor biology.[22,42,67] Furthermore, because this method is highly objective, most studies find a comparatively favorable interreader and intrareader agreement for SUV_{max}.[41,68] Probably as a result of

these properties, SUV_{max} is one of the most commonly used metrics for tumor viability[47] and, as previously shown, apparently has good prognostic properties in many tumor types.

However, studies into the reliability of SUV_{max} showed that this metric is biased in low count acquisitions; is sensitive to noise, tumor size, patient size, pixel size,[37,69] the reconstruction method and filter used (ie, the resolution of the image [ROI]),[38,68] and the scanner used[70]; and it has a comparatively worse test–retest reproducibility than SUV measures based on a larger ROI.[71] One explanation of the apparently strong correlation with survival may be that most studies were single-institution studies, which increases the consistency in subject preparation and scanner settings.

The authors believe that these studies showed the potential of metabolic metrics, but the frequent use of SUV_{max} should not necessarily lead to the

Table 1
Overview of studies in which tumor absorbed dose was correlated with outcome

Study	Number of Subjects (Lesions)	Device Type	Tumor Type	Metabolic Metric	Outcome
Flamen et al,[46] 2008	8 (39)	Resin	mCRC	TLG	TLG reduction >50% associated with significantly higher tumor absorbed dose
Eaton et al,[45] 2014	7 (30)	Resin	Metastatic melanoma	SUV_{max} TLG	Mean tumor dose correlates with change in SUV_{max} Maximum absorbed tumor dose correlates with decrease in TLG
van den Hoven et al,[35] 2016	30 (133)	Resin	mCRC	TLG	TLG reduction >50% predicts increased OS Significant dose–response relationship Dependence on baseline TLG found
Willowson et al,[65] 2017	22 (63)	Resin	mCRC	SUV_{peak} TLG	TLG reduction >65% associated with improved OS An average dose of 50 Gy was associated with TLG reduction >50%
Levillain et al,[66] 2018	24 (57)	Resin	mCRC	TLG	Average dose correlated with TLG reduction and increase in OS

conclusion that this is the best or most suited metric for response assessment.[48,72] For example, the utility and reliability of SUV_{max} in a multicenter setting is yet to be shown. The Positron Emission Tomography (PET) Response Criteria in Solid Tumors (PERCIST) criteria were explicitly formulated to encourage both improved test–retest reliability and standardization.[47] The development of user-friendly and validated software may aid in the adoption and standardization of more advanced metrics.[73]

Furthermore, there seems to be quite some variation in the implementation of metrics in the different studies, even within the same tumor type. This makes the direct pooling of standardized data and generalization of the results implausible. As a consequence, if there is to be an effort toward the articulation of formal guidelines, methods should be tested in a multicenter setting,[47,72] and subject preparation, scan, and analysis protocols should be harmonized across sites.[74–77]

SUMMARY

Due to its superior sensitivity, FDG-PET serves as a modality for tumor staging and visual detection of recurrence or disease progression. As such,

it is a reliable tool for patient selection and treatment management, also in radioembolization. Semiquantitative analysis of pretreatment metabolic uptake enables prognostication, which may further aid patient selection. Furthermore, the potential use of FDG-PET for treatment target volume delineation is described.

There is a lively ongoing discussion on metabolic response and whether it can serve as a more useful endpoint for clinical studies instead of morphologic metrics (eg, RECIST), which in many cases is a poor surrogate imaging endpoint.[10] The studies on radioembolization that have been reviewed here seem to support the notion that metabolic response is often exhibited earlier and correlates better with survival than anatomic response. This is a very important observation for research into the efficacy and, more currently, absorbed dose–response relationships of radioembolization. In the clinic, this enables earlier and more accurate treatment response monitoring and can aid changes in disease management.

However, there is some inconsistency in the metabolic response metrics that are used in the literature. Consequently, there is a great need for systematic studies with the aim to establish best practices and perhaps disease-specific metrics for the radioembolization paradigm. Such studies should aim to be compatible with guidelines on the standardization of patient preparation, scanner calibration, image acquisition, and analysis.

REFERENCES

1. Gibbs P, Gebski V, Van Buskirk M, et al. Selective Internal Radiation Therapy (SIRT) with yttrium-90 resin microspheres plus standard systemic chemotherapy regimen of FOLFOX versus FOLFOX alone as first-line treatment of non-resectable liver metastases from colorectal cancer: the SIRFLOX study. BMC Cancer 2014;14:897.

2. Dutton SJ, Kenealy N, Love SB, et al. FOXFIRE Protocol Development Group and the NCRI Colorectal Clinical Study Group. FOXFIRE protocol: an open-label, randomised, phase III trial of 5-fluorouracil, oxaliplatin and folinic acid (OxMdG) with or without interventional Selective Internal Radiation Therapy (SIRT) as first-line treatment for patients with unresectable liver-on. BMC Cancer 2014;14(5):497.

3. Van Hazel GA, Heinemann V, Sharma NK, et al. SIRFLOX: randomized phase III trial comparing first-line mFOLFOX6 (Plus or Minus Bevacizumab) versus mFOLFOX6 (Plus or Minus Bevacizumab) plus selective internal radiation therapy in patients with metastatic colorectal cancer. J Clin Oncol 2016;34(15):1723–31.

4. Wasan HS, Gibbs P, Sharma NK, et al. First-line selective internal radiotherapy plus chemotherapy versus chemotherapy alone in patients with liver metastases from colorectal cancer (FOXFIRE, SIRFLOX, and FOXFIRE-Global): a combined analysis of three multicentre, randomised, phase 3 trials. Lancet Oncol 2017;1159–71. https://doi.org/10.1016/S1470-2045(17)30457-6.

5. Vilgrain V, Pereira H, Assenat E, et al. Efficacy and safety of selective internal radiotherapy with yttrium-90 resin microspheres compared with sorafenib in locally advanced and inoperable hepatocellular carcinoma (SARAH): an open-label randomised controlled phase 3 trial. Lancet Oncol 2017; 18(12):1624–36.

6. Chow PKH, Gandhi M, Tan S-B, et al. SIRveNIB: selective internal radiation therapy versus sorafenib in Asia-Pacific patients with hepatocellular carcinoma. J Clin Oncol 2018. https://doi.org/10.1200/JCO.2017.76.0892.

7. Bastiaannet R, Kappadath SC, Kunnen B, et al. The physics of radioembolization. EJNMMI Phys 2018; 5(1):22.

8. Braat AJAT, Kappadath SC, Bruijnen RCG, et al. Adequate SIRT activity dose is as important as adequate chemotherapy dose. Lancet Oncol 2017; 18(11):e636.

9. Sposito C, Mazzaferro V. The SIRveNIB and SARAH trials, radioembolization vs. sorafenib in advanced HCC patients: reasons for a failure, and perspectives for the future. Hepatobiliary Surg Nutr 2018; 7(6):487–9.

10. Pinker K, Riedl C, Weber WA. Evaluating tumor response with FDG PET: updates on PERCIST, comparison with EORTC criteria and clues to future developments. Eur J Nucl Med Mol Imaging 2017; 44(S1):55–66.

11. Kennedy A, Nag S, Salem R, et al. Recommendations for radioembolization of hepatic malignancies using yttrium-90 microsphere brachytherapy: a consensus panel report from the radioembolization brachytherapy oncology consortium. Int J Radiat Oncol Biol Phys 2007;68(1):13–23.

12. Coldwell DM, Sangro B, Wasan HS, et al. General selection criteria of patients for radioembolization of liver tumors. Am J Clin Oncol 2011;34(3). https://doi.org/10.1097/COC.0b013e3181ec61bb.

13. Maffione AM, Lopci E, Bluemel C, et al. Diagnostic accuracy and impact on management of 18F-FDG PET and PET/CT in colorectal liver metastasis: a meta-analysis and systematic review. Eur J Nucl Med Mol Imaging 2015;42(1):152–63.

14. Kong G, Jackson C, Koh DM, et al. The use of 18F-FDG PET/CT in colorectal liver metastases—comparison with CT and liver MRI. Eur J Nucl Med Mol Imaging 2008;35(7):1323–9.

15. Rosenbaum CENM, van den Bosch MAAJ, Veldhuis WB, et al. Added value of FDG-PET imaging in the diagnostic workup for yttrium-90 radioembolisation in patients with colorectal cancer liver metastases. Eur Radiol 2013;23(4):931–7.

16. Denecke T, Rühl R, Hildebrandt B, et al. Planning transarterial radioembolization of colorectal liver metastases with Yttrium 90 microspheres: evaluation of a sequential diagnostic approach using radiologic and nuclear medicine imaging techniques. Eur Radiol 2008;18(5):892–902.

17. Schmidt GP, Paprottka P, Jakobs TF, et al. FDG–PET–CT and whole-body MRI for triage in patients planned for radioembolisation therapy. Eur J Radiol 2012;81(3):e269–76.

18. Yoon KT, Kim JK, Kim DY, et al. Role of ^{18}F-fluorodeoxyglucose positron emission tomography in detecting extrahepatic metastasis in pretreatment staging of hepatocellular carcinoma. Oncology 2007;72(1):104–10.

19. Bos BR, van Der Hoeven JJ, Van Der Wall E, et al. Biologic correlates of 18Fluorodeoxyglucose uptake in human breast cancer measured by positron emission tomography. J Clin Oncol 2002; 20(2):379–87.

20. Basu S, Zaidi H, Holm S, et al. Quantitative techniques in PET-CT imaging. Current Medical Imaging Reviews 2011;7(3):216–33.

21. Kole AC, Nieweg OE, Pruim J, et al. Standardized uptake value and quantification of metabolism for breast cancer imaging with FDG and L-[1-11C] tyrosine PET. J Nucl Med 1997;38(5):692–6. Available at: http://www.ncbi.nlm.nih.gov/pubmed/9170429.

22. Riedl CC, Akhurst T, Larson S, et al. 18F-FDG PET scanning correlates with tissue markers of poor prognosis and predicts mortality for patients after liver resection for colorectal metastases. J Nucl Med 2007;48(5):771–5.

23. Haug AR, Tiega Donfack BP, Trumm C, et al. 18F-FDG PET/CT predicts survival after radioembolization of hepatic metastases from breast cancer. J Nucl Med 2012;53(3):371–7.

24. Soydal C, Kucuk ON, Bilgic S, et al. Radioembolization with90Y resin microspheres for intrahepatic cholangiocellular carcinoma: prognostic factors. Ann Nucl Med 2016;30(1):29–34.

25. Eldredge-Hindy H, Ohri N, Anne PR, et al. Yttrium-90 microsphere brachytherapy for liver metastases from uveal melanoma. Am J Clin Oncol 2016;39(2):189–95.

26. Piduru SM, Schuster DM, Barron BJ, et al. Prognostic value of 18F-fluorodeoxyglucose positron emission tomography-computed tomography in predicting survival in patients with unresectable metastatic melanoma to the liver undergoing yttrium-90 radioembolization. J Vasc Interv Radiol 2012;23(7):943–8.

27. Sabet A, Ahmadzadehfar H, Bruhman J, et al. Survival in patients with hepatocellular carcinoma treated with 90Y-microsphere radioembolization. Nuklearmedizin 2014;53(2):39–45.

28. Abuodeh Y, Naghavi AO, Ahmed KA, et al. Prognostic value of pre-treatment F-18-FDG PET-CT in patients with hepatocellular carcinoma undergoing radioembolization. World J Gastroenterol 2016;22(47):10406–14.

29. Jreige M, Mitsakis P, Van Der Gucht A, et al. 18F-FDG PET/CT predicts survival after 90Y transarterial radioembolization in unresectable hepatocellular carcinoma. Eur J Nucl Med Mol Imaging 2017;44(7):1215–22.

30. Sun DW, An L, Wei F, et al. Prognostic significance of parameters from pretreatment18F-FDG PET in hepatocellular carcinoma: a meta-analysis. Abdom Radiol (NY) 2016;41(1):33–41.

31. Higashi K, Ueda Y, Ayabe K, et al. FDG PET in the evaluation of the aggressiveness of pulmonary adenocarcinoma: correlation with histopathological features. Nucl Med Commun 2000;21(8):707–14.

32. Brianzoni E, Rossi G, Ancidei S, et al. Radiotherapy planning: PET/CT scanner performances in the definition of gross tumour volume and clinical target volume. Eur J Nucl Med Mol Imaging 2005;32(12):1392–9.

33. Bradley J, Bae K, Choi N, et al. A phase II comparative study of gross tumor volume definition with or without PET/CT fusion in dosimetric planning for non–small-cell lung cancer (NSCLC): primary analysis of radiation therapy oncology group (RTOG) 0515. Int J Radiat Oncol Biol Phys 2012;82(1):435–41.e1.

34. Ho S, Lau WY, Leung TWT, et al. Partition model for estimating radiation doses from yttrium-90 microspheres in treating hepatic tumours. Eur J Nucl Med 1996;23(8):947–52.

35. van den Hoven AF, Rosenbaum CENM, Elias SG, et al. Insights into the dose-response relationship of radioembolization with resin 90Y-microspheres: a prospective cohort study in patients with colorectal cancer liver metastases. J Nucl Med 2016;57(7):1014–9.

36. Foster B, Bagci U, Mansoor A, et al. A review on segmentation of positron emission tomography images. Comput Biol Med 2014;50:76–96.

37. Boellaard R, Krak NC, Hoekstra OS, et al. Effects of noise, image resolution, and ROI definition on the accuracy of standard uptake values: a simulation study. J Nucl Med 2004;45(9):1519–27. Available at: http://jnm.snmjournals.org/content/45/9/1519.abstractN2 -.

38. Krak NC, Boellaard R, Hoekstra OS, et al. Effects of ROI definition and reconstruction method on quantitative outcome and applicability in a response monitoring trial. Eur J Nucl Med Mol Imaging 2005;32(3):294–301.

39. Bastiaannet R, van Roekel C, Kunnen B, et al. Is diffusion-weighted MRI really superior to PET/CT in predicting survival after radioembolization? Radiology 2018;289(1):274–5.

40. Shah B, Srivastava N, Hirsch AE, et al. Intra-reader reliability of FDG PET volumetric tumor parameters: effects of primary tumor size and segmentation methods. Ann Nucl Med 2012;707–14. https://doi.org/10.1007/s12149-012-0630-3.

41. Benz MR, Evilevitch V, Allen-Auerbach MS, et al. Treatment monitoring by 18F-FDG PET/CT in patients with sarcomas: interobserver variability of quantitative parameters in treatment-induced changes in histopathologically responding and nonresponding tumors. J Nucl Med 2008;49(7):1038–46.

42. Koksal D, Demirag F, Bayiz H, et al. The correlation of SUVmax with pathological characteristics of primary tumor and the value of Tumor/Lymph node SUVmax ratio for predicting metastasis to lymph nodes in resected NSCLC patients. J Cardiothorac Surg 2013;8(1). https://doi.org/10.1186/1749-8090-8-63.

43. Im H, Pak K, Cheon GJ, et al. Prognostic value of volumetric parameters of 18 F-FDG PET in non-small-cell lung cancer: a meta-analysis. Eur J Nucl

Med Mol Imaging 2015;241–51. https://doi.org/10.1007/s00259-014-2903-7.

44. Im HJ, Bradshaw T, Solaiyappan M, et al. Current methods to define metabolic tumor volume in positron emission tomography: which one is better? Nucl Med Mol Imaging 2018;52(1):5–15.

45. Eaton BR, Kim HS, Schreibmann E, et al. Quantitative dosimetry for yttrium-90 radionuclide therapy: tumor dose predicts fluorodeoxyglucose positron emission tomography response in hepatic metastatic melanoma. J Vasc Interv Radiol 2014;25(2):288–95.

46. Flamen P, Vanderlinden B, Delatte P, et al. Multimodality imaging can predict the metabolic response of unresectable colorectal liver metastases to radioembolization therapy with Yttrium-90 labeled resin microspheres. Phys Med Biol 2008;53(22):6591–603.

47. Wahl RL, Jacene H, Kasamon Y, et al. From RECIST to PERCIST: evolving considerations for PET response criteria in solid tumors. J Nucl Med 2009;50(Suppl_1):122S–50S.

48. Lammertsma AA. Forward to the past: the case for quantitative PET imaging. J Nucl Med 2017;58(7):1019–24.

49. Wong C, Salem R, Qing F, et al. Metabolic response after intraarterial 90Y-glass microsphere treatment for colorectal liver metastases: comparison of quantitative and visual analyses by 18F-FDG PET. J Nucl Med 2004;45:1892–7. Available at: http://onlinelibrary.wiley.com/o/cochrane/clcentral/articles/946/CN-00501946/frame.html.

50. Wong CYO, Qing F, Savin M, et al. Reduction of metastatic load to liver after intraarterial hepatic yttrium-90 radioembolization as evaluated by [18F] fluorodeoxyglucose positron emission tomographic imaging. J Vasc Interv Radiol 2005;16(8):1101–6.

51. Bienert M, McCook B, Carr BI, et al. 90Y Microsphere treatment of unresectable liver metastases: changes in 18F-FDG uptake and tumour size on PET/CT. Eur J Nucl Med Mol Imaging 2005;32(7):778–87.

52. Miller FH, Keppke AL, Reddy D, et al. Response of liver metastases after treatment with yttrium-90 microspheres: role of size, necrosis, and PET. Am J Roentgenol 2007;188(3):776–83.

53. Zerizer I, Al-Nahhas A, Towey D, et al. The role of early18F-FDG PET/CT in prediction of progression-free survival after90Y radioembolization: comparison with RECIST and tumour density criteria. Eur J Nucl Med Mol Imaging 2012;39(9):1391–9.

54. Shady W, Sotirchos VS, Do RK, et al. Surrogate imaging biomarkers of response of colorectal liver metastases after salvage radioembolization using 90y-loaded resin microspheres. Am J Roentgenol 2016;207(3):661–70.

55. Fendler WP, Philippe Tiega DB, Ilhan H, et al. Validation of several SUV-based parameters derived from 18F-FDG PET for prediction of survival after SIRT of hepatic metastases from colorectal cancer. J Nucl Med 2013;54(8):1202–8.

56. Sabet A, Meyer C, Aouf A, et al. Early post-treatment FDG PET predicts survival after 90Y microsphere radioembolization in liver-dominant metastatic colorectal cancer. Eur J Nucl Med Mol Imaging 2014;42(3):370–6.

57. Jongen JMJ, Rosenbaum CENM, Braat MNGJA, et al. Anatomic versus metabolic tumor response assessment after radioembolization treatment. J Vasc Interv Radiol 2018;29(2):244–53.e2.

58. Haug AR, Heinemann V, Bruns CJ, et al. 18F-FDG PET independently predicts survival in patients with cholangiocellular carcinoma treated with 90Y microspheres. Eur J Nucl Med Mol Imaging 2011;38(6):1037–45.

59. Camacho JC, Kokabi N, Xing M, et al. PET response criteria for Solid tumors predict survival at three months after intra-arterial resin-based 90Yttrium radioembolization therapy for unresectable intrahepatic cholangiocarcinoma. Clin Nucl Med 2014;39(11):944–50.

60. Michl M, Lehner S, Paprottka PM, et al. Use of PERCIST for prediction of progression-free and overall survival after radioembolization for liver metastases from pancreatic cancer. J Nucl Med 2016;57(3):355–60.

61. Wright CL, Binzel K, Zhang J, et al. Clinical feasibility of 90Y digital PET/CT for imaging microsphere biodistribution following radioembolization. Eur J Nucl Med Mol Imaging 2017;1–4. https://doi.org/10.1007/s00259-017-3694-4.

62. Carlier T, Willowson KP, Fourkal E, et al. 90 Y -PET imaging: exploring limitations and accuracy under conditions of low counts and high random fraction. Med Phys 2015;42(7):4295–309.

63. Willowson K, Forwood N, Jakoby BW, et al. Quantitative 90 Y image reconstruction in PET. Med Phys 2012;39(11):7153–9.

64. Gates VL, Esmail AAH, Marshall K, et al. Internal pair production of 90Y permits hepatic localization of microspheres using routine pet: proof of concept. J Nucl Med 2011;52(1):72–6.

65. Willowson KP, Hayes AR, Chan DLH, et al. Clinical and imaging-based prognostic factors in radioembolisation of liver metastases from colorectal cancer: a retrospective exploratory analysis. EJNMMI Res 2017;7(1):46.

66. Levillain H, Duran Derijckere I, Marin G, et al. 90Y-PET/CT-based dosimetry after selective internal radiation therapy predicts outcome in patients with liver metastases from colorectal cancer. EJNMMI Res 2018;8:1–9.

67. Lee DS, Kim SJ, Jang HS, et al. Clinical correlation between tumor maximal standardized uptake

value in metabolic imaging and metastatic tumor characteristics in advanced nonsmall cell lung cancer. Medicine (Baltimore) 2015;94(32):1–7.

68. Adams MC, Turkington TG, Wilson JM, et al. A systematic review of the factors affecting accuracy of SUV measurements. AJR Am J Roentgenol 2010;310–20. https://doi.org/10.2214/AJR.10.4923.

69. Lodge MA, Chaudhry MA, Wahl RL. Noise considerations for PET quantification using maximum and peak standardized uptake value. J Nucl Med 2012; 53(7):1041–7.

70. Kamibayashi T, Tsuchida T, Demura Y, et al. Reproducibility of semi-quantitative parameters in FDG-PET using two different PET Scanners: influence of attenuation correction method and examination interval. Mol Imaging Biol 2008;10(3):162–6.

71. Nahmias C, Wahl LM. Reproducibility of standardized uptake value measurements determined by 18F-FDG PET in malignant tumors. J Nucl Med 2008;49(11):1804–8.

72. Zaidi H, Alavi A, Naqa I El. Novel quantitative PET techniques for clinical decision support in oncology. Semin Nucl Med 2018. https://doi.org/10.1053/j.semnuclmed.2018.07.003.

73. Joo Hyun O, Wahl RL. PERCIST in perspective. Nucl Med Mol Imaging 2018;52(1):1–4.

74. Boellaard R, Delgado-Bolton R, Oyen WJG, et al. FDG PET/CT: EANM procedure guidelines for tumour imaging: version 2.0. Eur J Nucl Med Mol Imaging 2014;42(2):328–54.

75. Scheuermann JS, Saffer JR, Karp JS, et al. Qualification of PET scanners for use in multicenter cancer clinical trials: the American College of Radiology Imaging Network experience. J Nucl Med 2010;50(7): 1187–93.

76. Delbeke D, Coleman RE, Guiberteau MJ, et al. Procedure guideline for tumor imaging with 18F-FDG PET/CT 1.0. J Nucl Med 2006;47(5):885–95. Available at: http://jnm.snmjournals.org/content/47/5/885.long.

77. Aide N, Lasnon C, Veit-haibach P, et al. EANM/EARL harmonization strategies in PET quantification: from daily practice to multicentre oncological studies. Eur J Nucl Med Mol Imaging 2017;44:17–31.

Significant Value of ^{11}C-Acetate and ^{18}F-Fluorodeoxyglucose PET/Computed Tomography on ^{90}Y Microsphere Radioembolization for Hepatocellular Carcinoma

Chi Lai Ho, MD[a],*, Sirong Chen, PhD[a,b], Shing Kee Cheung, MBBS[a],
Thomas Wai Tong Leung, MD[c],*

KEYWORDS

- ^{90}Y microspheres • Radioembolization • HCC • ^{11}C-acetate • ^{18}F-FDG • PET/CT

KEY POINTS

- Pretreatment dual-tracer (^{18}F-FDG and ^{11}C-acetate) PET/CT has potential to predict treatment response for ^{90}Y microsphere radioembolization (RE) in patients with inoperable HCC. Patients with ^{11}C-acetate-avid HCC have a better response to ^{90}Y microsphere RE, and possibly better survival.
- Pretreatment dual-tracer PET/CT has a significant theranostic value on ^{90}Y microsphere RE in determining target tumor dose (TD) for HCC with different cellular differentiation, metabolic tumor volume, and functioning liver volume, and can be used to prescribe individual injected activity of ^{90}Y microspheres.
- Pretreatment tumor-to-nontumorous liver (T/NT) ratio of ^{99m}Tc-MAA has high accuracy in predicting post-treatment T/NT ratio of ^{90}Y microspheres, which determines the optimal balance between effective therapeutic radiation dose to tumors (TD) and risk to normal tissues (liver dose $\leq$70 Gy), an essential parameter in patient selection for the RE procedure.

INTRODUCTION

Hepatocellular carcinoma (HCC) is a primary malignancy of the hepatocyte, generally associated with an unfavorable prognosis.[1] It is the sixth most common cancer worldwide and the third leading cause of cancer mortality.[2] HCC frequently arises in the setting of cirrhosis (>80%) secondary to chronic hepatitis B or C, alcohol excess, and, increasingly, nonalcoholic fatty liver disease. Cirrhosis is a progressive process characterized by fibrosis and nodular disorder consisting in regenerative and dysplastic nodules, which have a propensity to transform into HCC. Patients who are at risk for HCC should undergo regular surveillance so that the cancers can be detected and treated during the early stage of development.

About 70% to 80% of patients with HCC do not qualify for a curative resection, transplantation, or radiofrequency ablation (RFA) because the diagnosis is often made either too late, at an advanced stage of the disease[3] or when hepatic functional

The authors declare no commercial or financial conflicts of interest and no funding sources.
[a] Department of Nuclear Medicine & PET, Hong Kong Sanatorium & Hospital, 2 Village Road, Happy Valley, Hong Kong, China; [b] Medical Physics & Research Department, Hong Kong Sanatorium & Hospital, 2 Village Road, Happy Valley, Hong Kong, China; [c] Comprehensive Oncology Center, Hong Kong Sanatorium & Hospital, 2 Village Road, Happy Valley, Hong Kong, China
* Corresponding authors.
E-mail addresses: garrettho@hksh.com (C.L.H.); Thomas.WT.Leung@hksh.com (T.W.T.L.)

reserve is too compromised to undergo a major operation. On the other hand, the 5-year tumor recurrence rate in these patients can sometimes be as high as 80%.[4]

For patients with inoperable HCC, palliative treatment as an option includes transarterial chemoembolization (TACE), RFA, percutaneous ethanol injection, microspheres radioembolization (RE), immunotherapy, and systemic chemotherapy. TACE is the most opted choice of therapy for the intermediate-stage HCC patients, and it has been shown to improve clinical outcomes and to serve as a bridging therapy to transplantation.[4,5] However, TACE is not applicable for patients with portal vein thrombosis (PVT). Although HCC is a radiosensitive tumor, the use of external beam radiation therapy is limited by a low threshold of radiation-induced hepatic toxicity to the normal liver cells. A dose of 30 Gy is typically designated as the dose of external beam irradiation that can induce hepatic damage.[6] However, this dose is insufficient to provide a treatment response to HCC tumors.

RE embedded with ^{90}Y microspheres is increasingly used for the treatment of inoperable HCC with or without PVT.[7–10] Intrahepatic malignancies derive the vast majority of their blood supply from the hepatic artery rather than the portal vein. Therefore, selective, catheter-based administration of ^{90}Y microspheres into the hepatic artery can deliver short-range radiation to the tumors, sparing normal liver parenchyma. ^{90}Y is a pure β-emitter with an average energy of 0.93 MeV. The mean penetration range is 2.5 mm in liver. Two commercially available forms of ^{90}Y are ^{90}Y-labeled glass (TheraSphere, BTG) and resin (SIR-Spheres; Sirtex) microspheres. ^{90}Y microspheres are much smaller than the TACE particles (20–60 μm vs 200–500 μm); therefore, the primary mechanism of ^{90}Y RE is through the radiation effect instead of embolic occlusion of tumor blood supply as takes place in TACE. Compared with external beam radiation, ^{90}Y RE allows delivery of a higher radiation dose of up to 50 to 150 Gy to the treated liver[11] and an even higher radiation dose of up to 100 to 1000 Gy to the tumor tissue.[12] Compared with TACE, it has been shown to bring longer progression-free survival (PFS), less toxicity, and increased quality of life to HCC patients.[13,14] Improved clinical outcome, from complete remission (CR) to partial remission, or stable disease, has been previously reported in 60% to 90% of cases.[15–17] It is also regarded as a bridging therapy for patients awaiting curative resection. Similar to other HCC treatments, the success rate of ^{90}Y microsphere RE depends highly on the ability of pretreatment imaging for accurate staging/restaging of patients' HCC disease status and the assessment of tumor burden and aggressiveness, which are all essential for prediction of treatment response and survival.[18–20] For ^{90}Y RE, understanding the cytokinetic logistics and principles behind the methodology and calculation of treatment dose to the tumors (TD) are especially important.[18] Dual-tracer, ^{11}C-acetate, and ^{18}F-fluorodeoxyglucose (FDG) PET/computed tomography (CT) has a proven role to play along the timeline of management for these patients.[18,21–25]

PRETREATMENT ^{11}C-ACETATE AND ^{18}F-FLUORODEOXYGLUCOSE PET/COMPUTED TOMOGRAPHY FOR STAGING OF HEPATOCELLULAR CARCINOMA, AND EVALUATION OF TUMOR BURDEN AND AGGRESSIVENESS

Accurate staging is important for selection of the most appropriate treatment approach for patients with HCC. Radiologic imaging in detection of HCC is based on a triphasic vascular pattern found on CT or MR imaging, typically with early arterial-contrast enhancement, followed by an isodense or hypodense appearance on portal venous phase with a persistent hypodensity on delayed phase. The sensitivity of radiologic imaging in the detection of HCC is less optimal in the presence of architectural distortion by severe cirrhosis, mostly reported as around 60% to 70%.[26,27] Some data have suggested that only about 10% to 30% of nodules measuring less than 2 cm seen on arterial phase of contrast CT imaging represent HCC in highly cirrhotic livers.[28] As a result, morphologic criteria alone are often insufficient for accurate staging and evaluation of tumor burden or tumor aggressiveness,[22,23] and would possibly compromise the selection of patients for the most appropriate treatment, as well as prediction of tumor recurrence risk and survival.[29]

Cytokinetic and pathologic factors known to affect prognosis include ^{18}F-FDG PET, tumor biology, histologic tumor grade, and microvascular invasion. In a retrospective study, Yang and colleagues[30] demonstrated that ^{18}F-FDG PET-positive patients showed an overall greater risk of tumor recurrence after liver transplantation (LT) compared with the ^{18}F-FDG PET–negative patients (odds ratio = 7.6). Kornberg and colleagues[31,32] demonstrated that ^{18}F-FDG uptake on PET is a reliable preoperative predictor of tumor recurrence after LT in patients with HCC, triggered by its high association with poor tumor differentiation and microvascular invasion. Therefore, patients with ^{18}F-FDG-avid HCC are often lower in priority on the transplant list. However, despite its prognostic value, ^{18}F-FDG PET has been shown to have a suboptimal sensitivity in detecting HCC. A high false-negative rate of 30% to 50% is primarily attributed to the underlying biochemistry of well to moderately differentiated HCC, which is not glycolysis dependent for tumor metabolism.[33–36]

The studies by Ho and colleagues[24,25] using a dual-tracer PET protocol comprising ^{18}F-FDG and ^{11}C-acetate have demonstrated that PET evaluation of HCC should be guided by the upregulated biochemistry of the tumor cells, which in turn depends on the degree of cellular differentiation of some types of tumors. Along the natural course of HCC disease development, the spectral changes in cellular differentiation and tumor aggressiveness may naturally necessitate a pair of complementary biochemical probes for more comprehensive evaluation of primary hepatic neoplasm. Whereas well-differentiated HCC has upregulated acetyl-coenzyme A synthase activity and shows increased avidity for ^{11}C-acetate, dedifferentiated HCC as a result of disease progression and increased aggressiveness is accompanied by changes in intracellular structure and biochemistry that prefers ^{18}F-FDG as main substrate. In general, ^{11}C-acetate is not found to be associated with poor prognostic indicators such as high tumor grade or microvascular invasion.[21] In a study by Cheung and Ho[22] on clinical staging and selection of HCC patients for LT, dual-tracer PET/CT had a high TNM staging accuracy in both LT and partial-hepatectomy groups of patients (90.9% vs 90.5%), significantly better than that of contrast CT (54.5% vs 28.6%). The use of dual-tracer PET/CT to select patients for LT is also significantly better than that of contrast CT (93.8% vs 43.8%), partly based on the findings that dual-tracer PET/CT is more accurate in evaluating the tumor burden in terms of number and size of HCC lesions. It has also shown that LT patients with HCC lesions purely avid for ^{11}C-acetate could achieve a significantly longer disease-free survival after LT (>80% at 5-year follow-up). In a study of 49 HCC patients with bone metastases,[37] ^{11}C-acetate PET/CT identified a special group of patients with isolated bone metastases, who had a significantly longer survival than other HCC patients with multiorgan metastases (median survival: 18 months vs 11 months). The ability of dual-tracer PET/CT in predicting treatment response and survival was also confirmed by Li and colleagues[23] in 22 patients treated with TACE and bevacizumab ($n = 11$) or placebo ($n = 11$). These investigators suggested that the collective utilization of individual molecular information (which reflects HCC cellular differentiation) provided by dual-tracer PET/CT might be useful in selecting the most effective therapy.

The role of ^{18}F-FDG PET/CT in patients with unresectable HCC undergoing ^{90}Y microspheres RE was also studied.[38,39] In a retrospective study of 33 patients,[38] ^{18}F-FDG–negative patients had a significantly longer overall survival (OS) than FDG-positive patients (13 months vs 9 months, $P = .010$). A recent study by Ho and colleagues[18] has demonstrated that HCC patients with lower tumor aggressiveness, as suggested by the tumor's avidity for the surrogate biomarker ^{11}C-acetate, might predict a better response to ^{90}Y microspheres RE (77% vs 27%) and a better 2-year OS than ^{18}F-FDG (86% vs 22%). In this study, treatment response was assessed 2 months after ^{90}Y glass microspheres RE by ^{11}C-acetate and ^{18}F-FDG PET/CT. A good responder was defined as having a post-treatment decrease of 50% or more compared with the pretreatment metabolic HCC tumor burden (MTB). MTB was defined as the "summation of the product of individual (lesion SUV_{mean}) × (lesion volume)" of all HCC lesions on ^{11}C-acetate or ^{18}F-FDG PET/CT.[40] A poor responder was defined as having an MTB decrease of less than 50% or having new HCC lesions after treatment. The incorporation of the metabolic index standardized uptake value (SUV) as well as metabolic volume into the calculation of MTB, instead of using the physical dimension(s) from CT/MR imaging, is based on a classic cytokinetic principle. It stipulates that a good biological parameter should reflect the tumor's true biological bulk and activity, and has the advantage of not including tumor necrosis or other nontumorous components that would otherwise be erroneously counted as tumor burden on structural imaging. **Fig. 1** shows a patient with HCC lesion purely avid for ^{11}C-acetate, indicating a well-differentiated HCC. He achieved CR after ^{90}Y glass microspheres RE, which was demonstrated on follow-up ^{11}C-acetate and ^{18}F-FDG PET/CT 2 months after treatment. This patient survived for more than 3 years. **Fig. 2** shows another patient with poorly differentiated HCC mainly avid by ^{18}F-FDG PET. He underwent ^{90}Y glass microspheres RE but follow-up PET/CT showed poor response to treatment by demonstrating only 40% reduction in MTB, and he died 9 months after therapy. Dual-tracer PET/CT was thus found to be useful to risk stratify the HCC patient and to select the appropriate candidates for individualized prescription of ^{90}Y microspheres RE.

PRESCRIPTION OF INJECTED ACTIVITY FOR ^{90}Y MICROSPHERE RADIOEMBOLIZATION

The success of ^{90}Y microspheres RE depends on optimization of the treatment dose of radionuclide particles distributed to the tumors while sparing

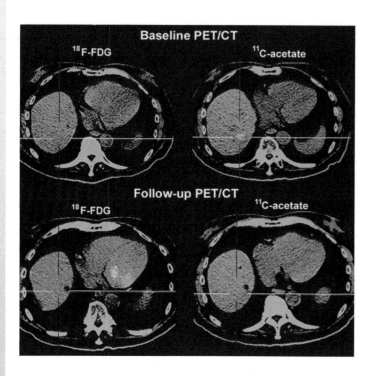

Fig. 1. On baseline PET/CT, the HCC lesion was purely ^{11}C-acetate-avid. After ^{90}Y glass microspheres RE, on follow-up PET/CT 2 months later, ^{11}C-acetate activity was normalized (100% reduction in MTB, complete remission). This patient was classified as a good responder. He survived for more than 3 years after ^{90}Y glass microspheres RE.

nontumorous liver (NTD) from radiation damage, as well as minimizing shunting to other organs.[41,42] Before treatment initiation, this approach requires a diagnostic angiography and a liver perfusion scan after intra-arterial injection of ^{99m}Tc-macro-aggregated albumin (^{99m}Tc-MAA) to assess the risk of extrahepatic deposition of microspheres and evaluate the percentage of lung shunting (S_{MAA}). MAA is chosen because of its similar physical size to ^{90}Y microspheres (20–50 μm). An arterial catheter is placed at the appropriate segment of the hepatic artery feeding the target lesion(s). Planning celiac and hepatic angiography is performed to define hepatic and tumor vascular anatomy. In particular, the hepatic artery and its branches supplying the tumors are identified.

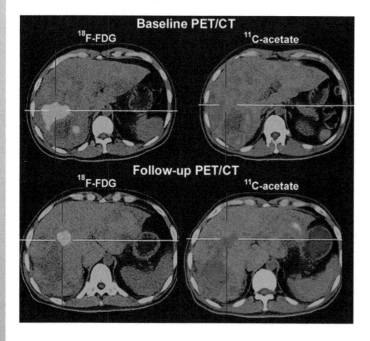

Fig. 2. On baseline PET/CT, the HCC lesions were primarily ^{18}F-FDG-avid. The patient underwent ^{90}Y glass microspheres RE within 2 weeks. On follow-up PET/CT 2 months after RE only 40% reduction in MTB was achieved, thus classifying the patient as a poor responder. This patient died 9 months after ^{90}Y glass microspheres RE.

Collateral arteries branching from the hepatic artery supplying the gallbladder, stomach, or intestine undergo coil embolization to avoid secondary complications. The presence of collateral arteries not amenable to coil embolization is considered a contraindication to ^{90}Y microspheres RE. The maximum permissible injected activity (IA) for each patient is first calculated by limiting the absorbed lung dose (LD) caused by shunting found on ^{99m}Tc-MAA scintigram to less than 30 to 35 Gy so as to avoid radiation pneumonitis.[43]

$$LD_{(Gy)} = IA_{(GBq)} \times S_{MAA} \times 49.67 \qquad (1)$$

where a lung mass of 1 kg is assumed, and 49.67 is the conversion factor of ^{90}Y from GBq/kg to Gy.

Dose delivered to the tumor (TD) is considered the most significant parameter of ^{90}Y RE in predicting the treatment response, PFS, and OS.[16,17,44–46] In a study of 36 patients with HCC, including 16 with PVT, Garin and colleagues[17] found that a threshold $T_{plan} D$ value of 205 Gy based on ^{99m}Tc-MAA single-photon emission CT (SPECT)/CT dosimetry is the only predictor of response and survival (14 months vs 18 months) in HCC patients treated with ^{90}Y glass microspheres. In 2014, Srinivas and colleagues[47] reported that among 56 patients being treated with ^{90}Y glass RE, the responders had received a mean dose of 215 Gy and the nonresponders 167 Gy based on post-RE ^{90}Y PET/CT dosimetry. However, the current standard dosimetry approach is to administer 120 ± 20 Gy (injected liver dose) to the treated liver containing the tumor(s), regardless of individual tumoral and nontumoral liver dosimetry. The IA of glass microspheres is determined by using the conventional Medical Internal Radiation Dose equation with adjustment of percentage of lung shunting (S_{MAA}) by pretreatment ^{99m}Tc-MAA scan.

$$IA_{(GBq)} = (120 \times 1.03 \times volume_{IL}) / ((1 - S_{MAA}) \times 49.67) \qquad (2)$$

where 1.03 kg/L is the liver/tumor density and volume$_{IL}$ is the volume of treated liver containing the tumor(s). Some centers apply a simplified 3-compartment (tumor, normal liver, and lung) algorithm to calculate the IA.[16,17,45,48–51] From the maximum permissible IA by the aforementioned lung shunting, dose reduction is adjusted according to the fractional tumor volume and ^{99m}Tc-MAA tumor-to-nontumor partition ratio (T/NT$_{MAA}$) under the condition that the normal liver absorbed dose must be less than 65 to 70 Gy.[10,45]

$$IA_{(GBq)} = (TD \times 1.03 \times volume_T + (TD/(T/NT_{MAA})) \times 1.03 \times volume_{NT}) / ((1 - S_{MAA}) \times 49.67) \qquad (3)$$

where volume$_T$ and volume$_{NT}$ are the volumes of tumor and functioning liver, respectively. Although more reasonable than the conventional dosimetry method, this 3-compartment protocol may have the following clinical/technical concerns:

- Is there a more accurate baseline imaging for the evaluation of HCC distribution, number of HCC tumors, and tumor volume (tumor burden)?
- What is the optimal TD to achieve good response to ^{90}Y RE treatment?
- Would the optimal TD for good response be different among various HCC grades of differentiation, given that abundant data in the literature have documented that there is a strong correlation between grades of cellular differentiation and treatment response, as well as PFS and OS?
- Can pretreatment ^{99m}Tc-MAA partition ratio (T/NT$_{MAA}$) correctly predict the ^{90}Y glass microspheres partition ratio (T/NT$_{90Y}$)?

On account of the first clinical concern, ^{11}C-acetate and ^{18}F-FDG PET/CT has already been shown to be an accurate imaging modality for the staging of HCC, evaluation of HCC tumor burden and tumor grade, and prediction of treatment response as well as survival. In an attempt to tackle the other concerns, a study of 62 patients with inoperable HCC[18] sought to investigate whether dual-tracer PET/CT had adequate power to determine the required TD in HCC with different cellular differentiation, so that better outcomes could be achieved with ^{90}Y RE. The investigators categorized the patients into 3 groups according to the metabolic information obtained from baseline ^{11}C-acetate and ^{18}F-FDG PET/CT:

- ^{11}C-acetate group (defined as having >70% tumor volume avid for ^{11}C-acetate as surrogate indicator of well-differentiated HCC)
- ^{18}F-FDG group (defined as having >70% tumor volume avid for ^{18}F-FDG as surrogate indicator of poorly differentiated HCC)
- Mixed group (avid for both tracers and not qualified as the first 2 groups, indicator of moderately differentiated HCC)

In this study,[18] ^{90}Y biodistribution was assessed directly by quantitative measurement of ^{90}Y PET/CT 17 to 22 hours after RE. Although the abundance of positron decay in ^{90}Y is intrinsically small (branching probability ratio of $[31.86 \pm 0.47] \times 10^{-6}$), it is nevertheless a direct method of confirmation and measurement of ^{90}Y activity. Like the majorities of studies on ^{90}Y PET/CT for dosimetry,[44,52,53] they also validated the feasibility of post-RE ^{90}Y PET/CT with a high recovery coefficient of 81.9% to

99.9% (mean = [92.7% ± 6.1%], median = 94.8%). In addition, they found a linear correlation ($T/NT_{90Y} = 1.01 \times T/NT_{MAA} + 0.161$, $r = 0.918$, $P \ll 0.05$) between post-treatment T/NT_{90Y} and pretreatment T/NT_{MAA}, allowing prediction of T/NT_{90Y} when calculating ^{90}Y prescription IA.

The same study[18] showed that by using 2 different PET tracers (^{11}C-acetate and ^{18}F-FDG) as metabolic surrogate markers of HCC cellular differentiation, the threshold ^{90}Y tumor doses (TD) to achieve good response are significantly different among them. ^{11}C-acetate-avid and mixed tumors (well and moderately differentiated HCC) require a target TD >152 Gy and >174 Gy, respectively, whereas the ^{18}F-FDG-avid tumors (poorly differentiated) require >262 Gy. These results of different dose requirements agree with the previous discussion that grades of cellular differentiation could affect treatment response to ^{90}Y RE. Therefore, ^{11}C-acetate-avid HCC requires less TD, and is more likely to have a good response to treatment, whereas ^{18}F-FDG-avid HCC needs an escalated TD to achieve a good response. Based on the achievement of tracer-specific TD and a maximum tolerated liver dose (NTD = 70 Gy), the lower limits of T/NT_{MAA} for patient selection of ^{90}Y RE are ^{11}C-acetate-avid HCC = 2.0, mixed HCC = 2.3, and ^{18}F-FDG-avid HCC = 3.5. With the tracer-specific TD, volume$_{-T}$, and volume$_{-NT}$ decided by pretreatment dual-tracer PET/CT, and T/NT_{90Y} predicted by pretreatment ^{99m}Tc-MAA simulation, prescription IA can be calculated by

$$IA_{(GBq)} = (TD \times 1.03 \times volume\_T \\ + (TD/(T/NT_{90Y})) \times 1.03 \\ \times volume\_NT/((1 - S_{MAA}) \times 49.67) \quad (4)$$

Fig. 3 illustrates a patient with poorly differentiated HCC having ^{18}F-FDG as the primary avid tracer (see **Fig. 3**A) on baseline dual-tracer PET/CT. The lesion margins are marked by mildly accentuated ^{11}C-acetate activities (see **Fig. 3**B) owing to neoproliferation of younger, well-differentiated HCC clones/generations along the periphery of the tumor. Pretreatment T/NT_{MAA} was 4.8, and thus the estimation of T/NT_{90Y} was 5.0. The target TD for this patient belonging to the ^{18}F-FDG group was set to be 270 Gy (>262 Gy), and the estimated NTD was 54 Gy (= 270/5.0, <70 Gy). Prescription IA for ^{90}Y treatment based on Equation (4) was 2.8 GBq. After RE, the patient was scanned by both ^{90}Y PET/CT (see **Fig. 3**C) and Bremsstrahlung-SPECT (see **Fig. 3**D). As the figure shows, the Bremsstrahlung-SPECT images are suboptimal in quality because of low photon yield and continuous X-ray spectrum, and are incapable of true dosimetric quantification. With ^{90}Y PET/CT,

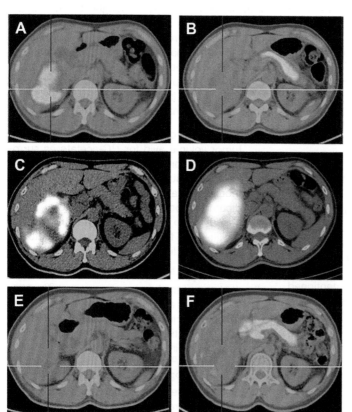

Fig. 3. A patient had a large inoperable HCC primarily avid for ^{18}F-FDG (*A*), categorized into the ^{18}F-FDG group. The lesion margin had mildly increased ^{11}C-acetate uptake (*B*). The planned TD of ^{90}Y glass microspheres RE was increased to 270 Gy. After RE, the patient was scanned by both ^{90}Y PET/CT (*C*) and Bremsstrahlung-SPECT (*D*). The latter has poor imaging quality and is incapable of true dosimetric quantification. ^{90}Y PET/CT dosimetry calculates a TD of 264 Gy, predicting a good responder. On follow-up ^{18}F-FDG (*E*) and ^{11}C-acetate (*F*) PET/CT 2 months after RE 90% reduction in MTB was achieved, thus confirming the patient as a good responder. This patient survived for more than 2 years after ^{90}Y glass microspheres RE.

however, direct dosimetry is possible, and the calculated TD was 264 Gy and NTD was 53 Gy (<70 Gy), predicting a good responder with little liver toxicity. On follow-up ^{18}F-FDG (see Fig. 3E) and ^{11}C-acetate (see Fig. 3F) PET/CT 2 months after RE, the patient achieved 90% reduction in MTB and was thus classified as a good responder. This patient survived for more than 2 years after ^{90}Y glass microspheres RE. This study also suggested an algorithm for the PET centers without ^{11}C-acetate PET based on Equation (4):

- Tumor and nontumor volumetry on ^{18}F-FDG PET/CT
- TD >262 Gy for ^{18}F-FDG-avid HCC (poorly differentiated), TD >174 Gy for non-^{18}F-FDG-avid HCC

Another observation from this study[18] was that the post–^{90}Y RE PET images of most of the patients had a metabolic biodistribution pattern resembling that of ^{11}C-acetate PET more than ^{18}F-FDG PET. It is speculated that poorly differentiated tumor cells often have a more blizzard-like growth environment, whereby a combination of hypoxia, necrosis, microvasculopathy, and tumor microthromboembolism could have caused disruption or impairment of proper ^{90}Y microsphere delivery to the tumor beds, resulting in a poor treatment response to ^{90}Y microspheres RE.

SUMMARY

Pretreatment dual-tracer (^{18}F-FDG and ^{11}C-acetate) PET/CT has a potential to predict treatment response for ^{90}Y microspheres RE in patients with inoperable HCC. Patients with ^{11}C-acetate-avid HCC have a better response to ^{90}Y microspheres RE, and possibly better survival, than patients with ^{18}F-FDG-avid HCC. Pretreatment dual-tracer PET/CT has a significant value in ^{90}Y microspheres RE regarding the decision of target TD for HCC with different cellular differentiation, metabolic tumor volume, and functioning liver volume, which can be used to calculate the individual IA of ^{90}Y microspheres. Pretreatment T/NT ratio of ^{99m}Tc-MAA predicts post-treatment T/NT ratio of ^{90}Y microspheres accurately, and is useful in selecting patients for RE based on the achievement of tracer-specific TD (related to HCC cellular differentiation) on the condition of liver dose ≤70 Gy.

REFERENCES

1. A new prognostic system for hepatocellular carcinoma: a retrospective study of 435 patients: the Cancer of the Liver Italian Program (CLIP) investigators. Hepatology 1998;28(3):751–5.

2. Ferlay J, Shin HR, Bray F, et al. Estimates of worldwide burden of cancer in 2008: GLOBOCAN 2008. Int J Cancer 2010;127(12):2893–917.

3. Bruix J, Sherman M, Llovet JM, et al. Clinical management of hepatocellular carcinoma. Conclusions of the Barcelona-2000 EASL conference. European Association for the Study of the Liver. J Hepatol 2001;35(3):421–30.

4. Llovet JM, Fuster J, Bruix J. The Barcelona approach: diagnosis, staging, and treatment of hepatocellular carcinoma. Liver Transpl 2004;10(2 Suppl 1):S115–20.

5. Bruix J, Sherman M. Management of hepatocellular carcinoma: an update. Hepatology 2011;53(3):1020–2.

6. Lewandowski RJ, Salem R. Yttrium-90 radioembolization of hepatocellular carcinoma and metastatic disease to the liver. Semin Intervent Radiol 2006; 23(1):64–72.

7. Salem R, Thurston KG. Radioembolization with ^{90}yttrium microspheres: a state-of-the-art brachytherapy treatment for primary and secondary liver malignancies. Part 1: technical and methodologic considerations. J Vasc Interv Radiol 2006;17(8): 1251–78.

8. Salem R, Thurston KG. Radioembolization with ^{90}yttrium microspheres: a state-of-the-art brachytherapy treatment for primary and secondary liver malignancies. Part 2: special topics. J Vasc Interv Radiol 2006;17(9):1425–39.

9. Salem R, Thurston KG. Radioembolization with yttrium-90 microspheres: a state-of-the-art brachytherapy treatment for primary and secondary liver malignancies: part 3: comprehensive literature review and future direction. J Vasc Interv Radiol 2006;17(10):1571–93.

10. Lau WY, Sangro B, Chen PJ, et al. Treatment for hepatocellular carcinoma with portal vein tumor thrombosis: the emerging role for radioembolization using yttrium-90. Oncology 2013;84(5):311–8.

11. Andrews JC, Walker SC, Ackermann RJ, et al. Hepatic radioembolization with yttrium-90 containing glass microspheres: preliminary results and clinical follow-up. J Nucl Med 1994;35(10):1637–44.

12. Kennedy AS, Nutting C, Coldwell D, et al. Pathologic response and microdosimetry of (90)Y microspheres in man: review of four explanted whole livers. Int J Radiat Oncol Biol Phys 2004;60(5): 1552–63.

13. Kulik LM, Carr BI, Mulcahy MF, et al. Safety and efficacy of ^{90}Y radiotherapy for hepatocellular carcinoma with and without portal vein thrombosis. Hepatology 2008;47(1):71–81.

14. Salem R, Lewandowski RJ, Mulcahy MF, et al. Radioembolization for hepatocellular carcinoma using Yttrium-90 microspheres: a comprehensive report of long-term outcomes. Gastroenterology 2010; 138(1):52–64.

15. Vente MA, Wondergem M, van der Tweel I, et al. Yttrium-90 microsphere radioembolization for the treatment of liver malignancies: a structured meta-analysis. Eur Radiol 2009;19(4):951–9.

16. Garin E, Rolland Y, Edeline J, et al. Personalized dosimetry with intensification using ^{90}Y-loaded glass microsphere radioembolization induces prolonged overall survival in hepatocellular carcinoma patients with portal vein thrombosis. J Nucl Med 2015;56(3): 339–46.

17. Garin E, Lenoir L, Rolland Y, et al. Dosimetry based on 99mTc-macroaggregated albumin SPECT/CT accurately predicts tumor response and survival in hepatocellular carcinoma patients treated with ^{90}Y-loaded glass microspheres: preliminary results. J Nucl Med 2012;53(2):255–63.

18. Ho CL, Chen S, Cheung SK, et al. Radioembolization with (90)Y glass microspheres for hepatocellular carcinoma: significance of pretreatment (11) C-acetate and (18)F-FDG PET/CT and posttreatment (90)Y PET/CT in individualized dose prescription. Eur J Nucl Med Mol Imaging 2018; 45(12):2110–21.

19. Kappadath SC, Mikell J, Balagopal A, et al. Hepatocellular carcinoma tumor dose response after (90)Y-radioembolization with glass microspheres using (90)Y-SPECT/CT-based voxel dosimetry. Int J Radiat Oncol Biol Phys 2018;102(2):451–61.

20. Jreige M, Mitsakis P, Van Der Gucht A, et al. (18)F-FDG PET/CT predicts survival after (90)Y transarterial radioembolization in unresectable hepatocellular carcinoma. Eur J Nucl Med Mol Imaging 2017;44(7): 1215–22.

21. Cheung TT, Chan SC, Ho CL, et al. Can positron emission tomography with the dual tracers [^{11}C]acetate and [^{18}F]fludeoxyglucose predict microvascular invasion in hepatocellular carcinoma? Liver Transplant 2011;17(10):1218–25.

22. Cheung TT, Ho CL, Lo CM, et al. ^{11}C-acetate and ^{18}F-FDG PET/CT for clinical staging and selection of patients with hepatocellular carcinoma for liver transplantation on the basis of Milan criteria: surgeon's perspective. J Nucl Med 2013;54(2): 192–200.

23. Li S, Peck-Radosavljevic M, Ubl P, et al. The value of [^{11}C]-acetate PET and [^{18}F]-FDG PET in hepatocellular carcinoma before and after treatment with transarterial chemoembolization and bevacizumab. Eur J Nucl Med Mol Imaging 2017;44(10):1732–41.

24. Ho CL, Yu SC, Yeung DW. ^{11}C-acetate PET imaging in hepatocellular carcinoma and other liver masses. J Nucl Med 2003;44(2):213–21.

25. Ho CL, Chen S, Yeung DW, et al. Dual-tracer PET/CT imaging in evaluation of metastatic hepatocellular carcinoma. J Nucl Med 2007;48(6):902–9.

26. Sangiovanni A, Manini MA, Iavarone M, et al. The diagnostic and economic impact of contrast imaging techniques in the diagnosis of small hepatocellular carcinoma in cirrhosis. Gut 2010;59(5): 638–44.

27. Yu NC, Chaudhari V, Raman SS, et al. CT and MRI improve detection of hepatocellular carcinoma, compared with ultrasound alone, in patients with cirrhosis. Clin Gastroenterol Hepatol 2011;9(2): 161–7.

28. Taouli B, Krinsky GA. Diagnostic imaging of hepatocellular carcinoma in patients with cirrhosis before liver transplantation. Liver Transpl 2006;12(11 Suppl 2):S1–7.

29. Lee JW, Paeng JC, Kang KW, et al. Prediction of tumor recurrence by ^{18}F-FDG PET in liver transplantation for hepatocellular carcinoma. J Nucl Med 2009; 50(5):682–7.

30. Yang SH, Suh KS, Lee HW, et al. The role of (18)F-FDG-PET imaging for the selection of liver transplantation candidates among hepatocellular carcinoma patients. Liver Transpl 2006;12(11):1655–60.

31. Kornberg A, Freesmeyer M, Barthel E, et al. ^{18}F-FDG-uptake of hepatocellular carcinoma on PET predicts microvascular tumor invasion in liver transplant patients. Am J Transplant 2009;9(3):592–600.

32. Kornberg A, Kupper B, Thrum K, et al. Increased ^{18}F-FDG uptake of hepatocellular carcinoma on positron emission tomography independently predicts tumor recurrence in liver transplant patients. Transplant Proc 2009;41(6):2561–3.

33. Delbeke D, Martin WH, Sandler MP, et al. Evaluation of benign vs malignant hepatic lesions with positron emission tomography. Arch Surg 1998;133(5):510–5 [discussion: 515–6].

34. Khan MA, Combs CS, Brunt EM, et al. Positron emission tomography scanning in the evaluation of hepatocellular carcinoma. J Hepatol 2000;32(5):792–7.

35. Okazumi S, Isono K, Enomoto K, et al. Evaluation of liver tumors using fluorine-18-fluorodeoxyglucose PET: characterization of tumor and assessment of effect of treatment. J Nucl Med 1992;33(3):333–9.

36. Trojan J, Schroeder O, Raedle J, et al. Fluorine-18 FDG positron emission tomography for imaging of hepatocellular carcinoma. Am J Gastroenterol 1999;94(11):3314–9.

37. Ho CL, Chen S, Cheng TK, et al. PET/CT characteristics of isolated bone metastases in hepatocellular carcinoma. Radiology 2011;258(2):515–23.

38. Sabet A, Ahmadzadehfar H, Bruhman J, et al. Survival in patients with hepatocellular carcinoma treated with 90Y-microsphere radioembolization. Prediction by ^{18}F-FDG PET. Nuklearmedizin 2014; 53(2):39–45.

39. Bagni O, Filippi L, Schillaci O. ^{18}F-FDG PET-derived parameters as prognostic indices in hepatic malignancies after ^{90}Y radioembolization: is there a role? Eur J Nucl Med Mol Imaging 2015; 42(3):367–9.

40. Wahl RL, Jacene H, Kasamon Y, et al. From RECIST to PERCIST: evolving considerations for PET response criteria in solid tumors. J Nucl Med 2009; 50(Suppl 1):122S–50S.

41. Pan CC, Kavanagh BD, Dawson LA, et al. Radiation-associated liver injury. Int J Radiat Oncol Biol Phys 2010;76(3 Suppl):S94–100.

42. Benson R, Madan R, Kilambi R, et al. Radiation induced liver disease: a clinical update. J Egypt Natl Canc Inst 2016;28(1):7–11.

43. Ho S, Lau WY, Leung TW, et al. Clinical evaluation of the partition model for estimating radiation doses from yttrium-90 microspheres in the treatment of hepatic cancer. Eur J Nucl Med 1997;24(3):293–8.

44. Kao YH, Steinberg JD, Tay YS, et al. Post-radioembolization yttrium-90 PET/CT—part 2: dose-response and tumor predictive dosimetry for resin microspheres. EJNMMI Res 2013;3(1):57.

45. Garin E. Radioembolization with (90)Y-loaded microspheres: high clinical impact of treatment simulation with MAA-based dosimetry. Eur J Nucl Med Mol Imaging 2015;42(8):1189–91.

46. Lam MG, Banerjee A, Goris ML, et al. Fusion dual-tracer SPECT-based hepatic dosimetry predicts outcome after radioembolization for a wide range of tumour cell types. Eur J Nucl Med Mol Imaging 2015;42(8):1192–201.

47. Srinivas SM, Natarajan N, Kuroiwa J, et al. Determination of radiation absorbed dose to primary liver tumors and normal liver tissue using post-radioembolization (90)Y PET. Front Oncol 2014;4:255.

48. Chiesa C, Mira M, Maccauro M, et al. A dosimetric treatment planning strategy in radio-embolization of hepatocarcinoma with ^{90}Y glass microspheres. Q J Nucl Med Mol Imaging 2012; 56(6):503–8.

49. Ho S, Lau WY, Leung TW, et al. Partition model for estimating radiation doses from yttrium-90 microspheres in treating hepatic tumours. Eur J Nucl Med 1996;23(8):947–52.

50. Ho S, Lau WY, Leung TW, et al. Tumour-to-normal uptake ratio of ^{90}Y microspheres in hepatic cancer assessed with 99Tcm macroaggregated albumin. Br J Radiol 1997;70(836):823–8.

51. Cao X, He N, Sun J, et al. Hepatic radioembolization with yttrium-90 glass microspheres for treatment of primary liver cancer. Chin Med J (Engl) 1999; 112(5):430–2.

52. Kao YH, Steinberg JD, Tay YS, et al. Post-radioembolization yttrium-90 PET/CT—part 1: diagnostic reporting. EJNMMI Res 2013;3(1):56.

53. Willowson KP, Tapner M, QUEST IT, et al. A multicentre comparison of quantitative (90)Y PET/CT for dosimetric purposes after radioembolization with resin microspheres : the QUEST Phantom Study. Eur J Nucl Med Mol Imaging 2015;42(8): 1202–22.

PET/CT Specificities in ^{90}Y Imaging Post Radioembolization

Walrand Stephan, PhD*, Hesse Michel, PhD

KEYWORDS

- Yttrium-90 • PET • Liver radioembolization • Quantification • Dosimetry

KEY POINTS

- ^{90}Y PET imaging does not require dedicated noise filtering using two 20-minute bed positions.
- Observed heterogeneities contain relevant dosimetry information.
- TOF has a major impact in extrahepatic sphere delivery exclusion.
- Valuable ^{90}Y PET-based dose-response predictions were verified.

INTRODUCTION

^{90}Y imaging appeared early in the genesis of nuclear medicine: the first ^{90}Y bremsstrahlung imaging was already that of a liver post radioembolization with ^{90}Y-loaded 15-μm-diameter microspheres and was performed in 1966 by Simon and colleagues[1,2] using a rectilinear scanner. Paradoxically, despite this long history, ^{90}Y is still nowadays a radionuclide whose imaging benefits from constant innovations, such as the first ^{90}Y TOF PET imaging in human performed in the authors' laboratory in 2009.[3] This PET acquisition was initiated by a micro-Derenzo phantom PET imaging made in 2004 by Nickles and colleagues,[4] itself based on a theoretic discovery elaborated in 1955 by Ford.[5] The fact that the 2 first images in humans dealt with liver radioembolization, both in an epoch where this act represented a small part of ^{90}Y medical applications, emphasizes the importance of ^{90}Y imaging for this therapeutic exploit.

Following the first ^{90}Y PET/CT imaging in humans, the impact of reconstruction parameters on tumor dose assessment after radioembolization has been intensely investigated in phantom studies.[6–16] Noise and contrast recovery were assessed for various sphere diameters, or vial sizes, filled with homogeneous activity simulating

tumors and set in a homogenous active background simulating healthy parenchyma. The background volumes ranged from 1- to 6-fold that of a normal liver. The specific activity ratio between spheres and background ranged from 4 to 8. These huge variations in phantom setups resulted in a large range of optimal reconstruction parameters: 1 up to 3 iterations × 21 subsets, with or without Gaussian postfiltering.

Comparison of ^{90}Y bremsstrahlung single-photon emission computed tomography (SPECT) and ^{90}Y PET was also evaluated in 4 studies,[17–20] all of which concluded that PET provided better spatial resolution and quantification accuracy than bremsstrahlung SPECT using a parallel-holes collimator.

Several dose-response relationships were reported using PET/CT-based tumor dosimetry.[21–25] The first one showed that, as in external beam radiotherapy, the baseline hemoglobin significantly affects the irradiation efficacy.[21] This was later confirmed in a large 600-patient series.[26] All the observed ^{90}Y PET-based dose-response relations confirmed the factor 2 already observed in the bremsstrahlung SPECT studies between the glass and resin microsphere efficacy per Gray.[27,28]

This article aims to provide a comprehensive review of the specific challenges inherent to ^{90}Y PET imaging, which should help in designing the

Nuclear Medicine, Cliniques Universitaires Saint-Luc, Avenue Hippocrate 10, 1200 Brussels, Belgium
* Corresponding author.
E-mail address: stephan.walrand@uclouvain.be

PET Clin 14 (2019) 469–476
https://doi.org/10.1016/j.cpet.2019.06.001

appropriate practice in phantom evaluation, as well as in postradioembolization dosimetry and sphere-delivery checks.

QUANTIFICATION OF INTRAHEPATIC ACTIVITY

Strydhorst and colleagues[29] modeled by Monte Carlo (MC) the acquisition of the NEMA PET phantom (NU2-1994) with one insert filled with ^{90}Y. **Fig. 1A** shows the simulated count-rate contribution of the different kinds of coincidences.

The ^{90}Y positron branching factor producing the 2 511-keV γ-rays is 0.0032%.[30] Bremsstrahlung x-rays are emitted with a continuous energy spectrum extending up to 2.3 MeV, corresponding to an abundance per decay of $\approx$0.14% in the PET acquisition energy window.[31] Consequently, the major part of the randoms involving 1 (g in **Fig. 1**) or 2 (f in **Fig. 1**) ^{90}Y decays arises from the x-ray contributions, resulting in a random fraction much higher than in pure positron emitter acquisitions. In addition, for PET systems based on Lu crystals, the randoms originating from the crystal's natural radioactivity (h in **Fig. 1**) dramatically worsen the random fraction as a result of the low positron abundance.

In comparison with pure positron emitters, such as ^{18}F, ^{90}Y exhibits additional disturbing true spurious coincidences between 2 x-rays (c in **Fig. 1**) or even from one single high-energy x-ray producing an e+e-pair creation, mainly in the dense crystal (d in **Fig. 1**). Another kind of spurious coincidence was not listed in **Fig. 1**, namely true coincidence between one 511-keV γ-ray and one x-ray, both originating from the same ^{90}Y decay. However, all these spurious coincidence contributions have a low occurrence and thus have a negligible impact on the activity quantification.[29]

Contrary to ^{124}I and ^{86}Y in which spurious coincidences are abundant,[32,33] no special correction is needed for ^{90}Y time-of-flight (TOF) PET quantitative imaging of targets large enough to avoid partial volume effect.[30] The situation is similar for non-TOF PET, apart from the fact that old bismuth germanate (BGO) PET studies evidenced dead time issues at greater than 1 GBq owing to the abundant x-rays,[7] although a study using a recent BGO PET has not verified this issue.[34] Dead time has thus to be investigated when using a BGO system before carrying out ^{90}Y quantitative PET imaging post liver radioembolization.

On the other hand, **Fig. 1A** clearly shows that noise in reconstructed images could be an issue,

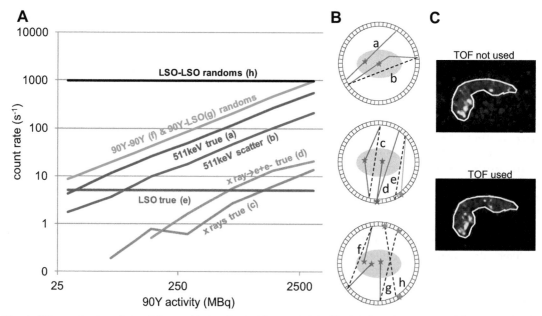

Fig. 1. (*A*) count rates of the different kinds of coincidences (cc) in ^{90}Y PET imaging extracted from MC simulations performed by Strydhorst and colleagues.[29] (*B*) Schematic representation of these coincidences (*red lines*: 511-keV γ-rays; *violet lines*: x-rays; *blue line*: ^{176}Lu γ-rays; red star: ^{90}Y decay; blue star: ^{176}Lu decay; brown star: e+e-pair creation). a: useful 511 keV true cc; b: 511-keV scattered cc; c: true cc between 2 x-rays; d: true cc originating from the e+e-pair creation in the crystal by a high-energy x-ray; e: true cc from one ^{176}Lu decay; f: random cc between 2 bremsstrahlung x-rays. g: random cc between a γ-ray or an x-ray with a Lu-based crystal decay; h: random cc between 2 ^{176}Lu decays. (*C*) LYSO PET imaging post liver radioembolization with or without the TOF information.

given that most of the recorded prompt coincidences are randoms. One has to keep in mind that if the randoms produced by [176]Lu are not present when using BGO PET, the x-rays randoms rate is increased by a factor of ≈ 4 because of the larger coincidence time window imposed by the slower scintillation light decay of BGO.[7]

EXTRAHEPATIC SPHERES DELIVERY CHECK

The spurious extrahepatic counts (see **Fig.** 1C) often observed in ^{90}Y non-TOF PET imaging using Lu-based crystal detectors result from the failure of conventional random correction to avoid positive bias in low-count-rate studies.[35] These residual counts are artificially magnified by the attenuation correction implemented in the reconstruction. Mathematics has proved that TOF reconstruction has a better robustness against emission-transmission inconsistencies. This property avoids such artificial magnification,[35] resulting in imaging free of spurious extrahepatic counts (see **Fig.** 1C).

PARTIAL VOLUME EFFECT

Willowson and colleagues[13] conducted a multi-center comparison of ^{90}Y quantitative imaging using a wide panel of PET/CT systems. The 9.6-L NEMA IEC PET body phantom (NU2-2001) was filled with 3 GBq with a hot-sphere-to-background contrast ratio of 8. Hot-sphere activities were measured using a spherical volume of interest (VOI) with the actual sphere diameter. **Fig.** 2 summarizes the results obtained by the 3 major manufacturers using their nondigital Lu-based crystal systems. **Fig.** 2 shows that, in this challenging low-specific-activity phantom, the impact of TOF information is more important than that of point spread function (PSF) correction. These results also clearly showed the additional benefit of taking into account the system PSF in TOF reconstruction (not commercially available for the PET system represented in blue, and not discardable for the PET represented in green).

Van Elmbt and colleagues[7] performed a comparison of 3 PET systems without PSF compensation (the one represented in blue in **Fig.** 2, one BGO PET, and one GSO PET). The phantom was a 3.6-L 20-cm-diameter cylinder phantom filled with 1.6 GBq and containing the hot spheres, with a contrast of 3 versus the background. Here, too, the study demonstrated the major impact of TOF. To reduce the partial volume effect, this study used the simple post correction,

$$A_{sph}^{corr} = A_{bg} + \frac{A_{sph} - A_{bg}}{RC} \quad (1)$$

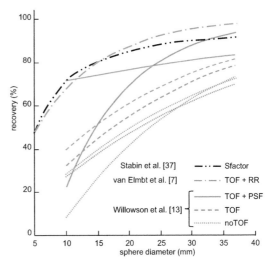

Fig. 2. Blue, brown, and green curves: fit ($y = 100 - ae^{-bx}$) of the hot spheres recovery as a function of the diameter for 3 different TOF PET systems. Solid, dashed, and dotted lines: fits of graphs a–f in **Fig. 4** from Willowson and colleagues.[13] Dash-dotted line: fit of TOF contrast in Fig. 6 from van Elmbt and coleagues.[7] Each color corresponds to a specific Lu-based crystal PET system. Solid and dotted lines correspond to TOF reconstruction taking into account the system PSF, while the dash-dotted line corresponds to a TOF reconstruction without PSF compensation, afterward corrected using Equation (1). Black curve: energy fraction delivered inside the sphere for a uniform ^{90}Y intrasphere distribution, computed using the spheres module in OLINDA.[37]

where the specific sphere activity A_{sph} was measured using a spherical VOI with the same diameter as the sphere, and the background specific activity A_{bg} using a shell VOI surrounding the sphere. RC is the theoretic recovery coefficient[36] corresponding to the system spatial resolution measured on a ^{90}Y point source. **Fig.** 2 shows that the corrected sphere recovery (dash-dotted line) is as good to that obtained using TOF PET with PSF compensation available in the 2 other TOF PET systems (solid lines).

INTRAHEPATIC SIGNAL-TO-NOISE RATIO

A common and useful tool to evaluate the signal-to-noise ratio (SNR) in PET is the well-known noise equivalent counts (NEC), defined as

$$NEC = \frac{T^2}{T+S+R} \quad (2)$$

where T, S, and R are the true, the scatter, and the random coincidences, respectively.

Strother and colleagues[38] and Conti[39] made very interesting improvements to Equation (2) in order to take into account the different methods of randoms correction and the TOF information, respectively. Combination of both improvements results in

$$SNR^2 \approx \frac{4}{\pi} \left(\frac{d}{D}\right)^3 \frac{D}{\min(D,\Delta)} \frac{T^2}{T+S+\nu\,(D/D_{FOV})^n\,R} \quad (3)$$

where D is the diameter of the active object to be imaged, d is the reconstruction voxel size, D_{FOV} is the system field-of-view diameter, and Δ is the positional uncertainty caused by TOF resolution. The parameter ν depends on the method used to correct for the randoms: it is set to 2 in case of direct random subtraction and to 1 when using variance reduction techniques to estimate the random distribution.

The parameter n is set to 1 or 2 for non-TOF and TOF systems, respectively. Indeed, randoms have a uniform distribution; thus for non-TOF PET only the random fraction with a line of response (LOR) crossing the object has an impact on the object imaging, that is, D/D_{FOV}. In addition, for a TOF PET only, the randoms having a TOF corresponding to the LOR segment contained in the object have an impact, resulting in a final fraction $(D/D_{FOV})^2$. Similarly to the conventional NEC, this SNR estimation is mainly based on a geometric analysis of the counts partition in the reconstructed image. It has the limitation of neglecting the tomographic ill-posed nature and the transmission-emission inconsistency, as discussed in the section on checking the delivery of extrahepatic spheres.

Equation (3) shows that TOF information improved the SNR via 2 terms: (1) $D/\min(D, \Delta)$, which increases when the TOF resolution improves, and (2) $(D/D_{FOV})^n$, which still decreases the impact of randoms as n reaches 2. Compared with a conventional PET, the first term provides an SNR improvement factor of ≈ 1.4 when using a 500-ps TOF PET system in liver lobe radioembolization.

Equation (3) teaches us other important features too. Current TOF PET crystals contain natural radioactivity giving a constant random rate. Thus for the same total true counts T, the randoms fraction will be larger when imaging a lower activity (even for a longer acquisition time), resulting in a lower SNR. Moreover, for the same total activity, the SNR will be lower if the activity is distributed in a larger volume. These 2 features imply that phantom validations have to use an activity distribution similar to that of the modeled clinical situation.

Fig. 3 illustrates the SNR obtained using Equation (3) for different systems as a function of the total activity located inside a volume of 20 cm diameter. One can clearly see the positive impact of the TOF information and, with a lower magnitude, of the kind of randoms correction ($\nu = 1$ or $\nu = 2$). Note the SNR saturation of the slower BGO crystal PET resulting from its larger coincidence time window, which increases randoms counts originating from the x-rays.[7]

The vertical red line in **Fig. 3A** corresponds to a typical liver radioembolization activity. This situation was modeled by van Elmbt and colleagues[7] using a hot-spheres phantom (**Fig. 3B**), in which the background volume was reduced to approach that of a liver. The hot-spheres specific activity was 3-fold that of the background. One can see that the relative visual quality of the images is in agreement with the predicted SNR. The worse image was obtained by the LYSO PET without using the TOF information as a result of the randoms originating from the LYSO natural radioactivity. This contribution is much larger than the true counts (see **Fig. 1A**) as a consequence of the low positron ^{90}Y branching factor. Using TOF information, the LYSO PET provided the best image. As discussed earlier, the acquisition of the phantom after 2 ^{90}Y half-lives results in a lower SNR (brown dashed curve) despite the increase in the acquisition time by a factor 4.

INTRAHEPATIC HETEROGENEITY PATTERN

In typical ^{90}Y imaging post liver radioembolization, the TOF PET system reached an SNR of about 2 (red line in **Fig. 3A**). Equation 2 applied to a typical liver imaging post fluorodeoxyglucose (FDG) injection with the same TOF-PET[40] gives a similar SNR. This similarity appears quite amazing because the ^{18}F positron abundance is about 3000-fold higher than that of ^{90}Y. The explanation is that ^{18}F activity and acquisition time in liver 1 hour post FDG injection are about 80- and 30-fold lower than those in ^{90}Y post liver radioembolization, respectively.

MC simulation of sphere transport in the hepatic arterial tree[41–43] showed that the sphere distribution has a heterogeneity pattern similar to that of the reconstructed activity (**Fig. 4A,B**), linked to the fact that the number of spheres (50–2500 Bq/sphere) is only one order of magnitude higher than the number of hepatic triad arteries. In contrast, the number of FDG molecules (10^{-4} Bq/molecule) metabolized by the liver is about 3 orders of magnitude higher than the accumulation of spheres. This huge number dramatically dumps the random spatial fluctuations in FDG liver activity.

A similar heterogeneity pattern is observed in liver tissue biopsies post ^{90}Y sphere radioembolization[44–46] (**Fig. 4C**) and in high-resolution MR

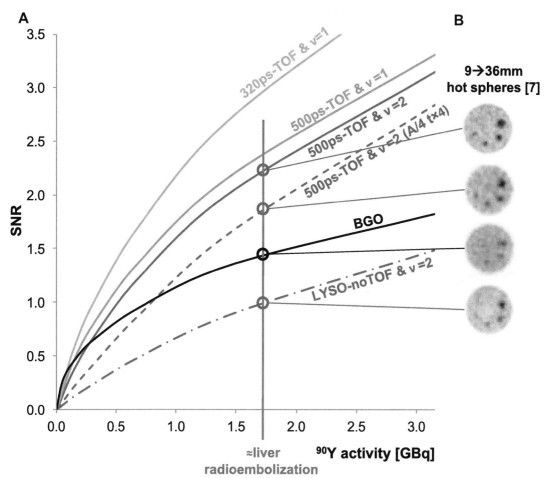

Fig. 3. (*A*) SNR estimations as a function of the total ^{90}Y activity derived from Equation (1) for a 20 minutes acquisition time *t* and using the different coincidences contributions computed for a 20-cm-diameter phantom with MC by Strydhorst and colleagues.[29] The dashed brown line corresponds to an acquisition with a specific activity 4-fold lower associated with an acquisition time of 80 minutes to keep the same total number of ^{90}Y decays. The BGO curve was approximated by leaving out the contribution h and e of **Fig. 2**, by rescaling the ^{90}Y randoms by a factor of 4 while the scatter fraction was extracted from van Elmbt and colleagues.[7] (*B*) Images obtained for the phantom used in van Elmbt and colleagues,[7] which corresponds to a typical liver radioembolization with a hot-sphere-to-background specific ratio of 3.

images post ^{166}Ho liver radioembolization[47] (**Fig. 4**D). Recently (**Fig. 4**E), unfiltered ^{90}Y TOF PET-based equivalent uniform dosing (EUD) has been shown to reunify patient survival prediction after resin and glass sphere radioembolization of hepatocellular carcinoma.[48]

All these facts show that there is no rationale for oversmooth liver ^{90}Y PET imaging post radioembolization in order to mimic the homogeneity observed in FDG liver PET imaging of the same patient.

SUMMARY
Phantom Validation

Phantom validation of ^{90}Y PET imaging intended for clinical ^{90}Y treatment assessment should be performed using activity, volume of distribution, and acquisition time similar to those used for clinical treatment.

Activity Quantification

No special correction is needed for activity quantification in large targets. For tumors, a compensation of the system PSF is required, that is, implementation of the system PSF in the reconstruction algorithm or post tumor activity correction, using Equation (1) with the system spatial resolution measured on a ^{90}Y point source. Both methods limit the underestimation of the activity to −20% and −50% for tumors larger than 25 mm when using a TOF PET or a non-TOF PET, respectively.

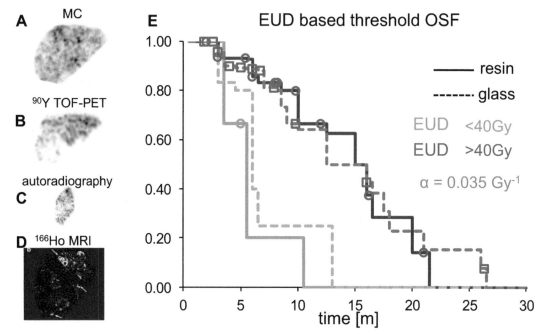

A MC

B ⁹⁰Y TOF-PET

autoradiography
C

D ¹⁶⁶Ho MRI

E EUD based threshold OSF

—— resin
------ glass

EUD <40Gy
EUD >40Gy
α = 0.035 Gy⁻¹

time [m]

Fig. 4. (A) Sphere-deposition simulation by MC.[41,42] (B) Typical ⁹⁰Y TOF PET unfiltered imaging post radioembolization. (C) Autoradiograph of excised liver piece post radioembolization. (D) MRI imaging post ¹⁶⁶Ho radioembolization. (E) Patient overall survival fraction (OSF). ([A] *Data from* Walrand S, Hesse M, Chiesa C, Lhommel R, Jamar F. The low hepatic toxicity per Gray of ⁹⁰Y glass microspheres is linked to their transport in the arterial tree favoring a nonuniform trapping as observed in posttherapy PET imaging. J Nucl Med 2014;5:135–40; and Walrand S. Microsphere deposition, dosimetry, radiobiology at the cell-scale, and predicted hepatic toxicity. In Handbook of radioembolization, physics, biology, nuclear medicine, and imaging. Pasciak AS, McKinney JM, Bradley YC (eds). Taylor & Francis. Boca Raton, FL. CRC Press 2016; [C] Courtesy of P. Bernhardt, Gothenburg, Sweden; [D] *Courtesy of* GEH Lam, Utrecht, the Netherlands; [E] *From* d'Abadie P, Hesse M, Jamar F, Lhommel R, Walrand S. ⁹⁰Y TOF-PET based EUD reunifies patient survival prediction in resin and glass microspheres radioembolization of HCC tumours. Phys Med Biol 2018;63:245010; with permission.)

When more accurate results are needed, the tumor activity should be corrected using Equation (1) with the RC derived from **Fig. 2**, or from an equivalent curve obtained for the considered PET system.

Old BGO PET systems can exhibit uncorrectable dead time issues at values greater than 1 GBq. For quantitative imaging, the user has to check (eg, in the literature or by phantom acquisitions) whether this is the case for the considered BGO PET system.

Dosimetry Assessment

Fig. 2 shows that even with compensation of the theoretic system PSF, the sphere recovery (solid and dash-dotted colored curves) is lower, or similar to, the energy fraction delivered in the sphere uniformly filled with ⁹⁰Y (black curve). As a result, the dose should be computed using

$$D = 50 \frac{A}{M} \qquad (4)$$

where M (kg) and A (Gy) are the mass and the activity in the considered target (eg, tumor, voxel, kidney, liver), respectively. This dose calculation,

called the local deposition method, has already been proposed and proved accurate.[11,28,49–52]

SNR computation, MC simulation, liver biopsies, and ¹⁶⁶Ho MR imaging clearly support that the intrahepatic heterogeneity observed in ⁹⁰Y PET post radioembolization imaging is mainly related to the actual sphere-distribution heterogeneity and thus should not be smoothened using an additional filter, especially when computing the EUD.[48]

Two 20-minute bed positions are required to obtain an SNR similar to that obtained in liver imaging after FDG injection.

Spheres Delivery Check

The clinician has to be aware that low spurious extrahepatic activity can be seen using Lu crystal-based non-TOF PET, which could make the task difficult.

REFERENCES

1. Simon N, Feitelberg S, Warner RRP, et al. External scanning of internal beta-emitters. J Mt Sinai Hosp N Y 1966;33:365–70.

2. Simon N, Feitelberg S. Scanning bremsstrahlung of yttrium-90 microspheres injected intra-arterially. Radiology 1967;88:719–24.

3. Lhommel R, Goffette P, Van den Eynde M, et al. Yttrium-90 TOF PET scan demonstrates high-resolution biodistribution after liver SIRT. Eur J Nucl Med Mol Imaging 2009;36(10):1969.

4. Nickles RJ, Roberts AD, Nye JA, et al. Assaying and PET imaging of yttrium-90: 1>>34 ppm>0. IEEE Nucl Sci Symp Conf Rec 2004;6:3412–4.

5. Ford K. Predicted 0+ level of Zr90. Phys Rev 1955; 98:1516.

6. Lhommel R, van Elmbt L, Goffette P, et al. Feasibility of ^{90}Y TOF PET-based dosimetry in liver metastasis therapy using SIR-Spheres. Eur J Nucl Med Mol Imaging 2010;37:1654–62.

7. van Elmbt L, Vandenberghe S, Walrand S, et al. Comparison of yttrium-90 quantitative imaging by TOF and non-TOF PET in a phantom of liver selective internal radiotherapy. Phys Med Biol 2011;56:6759.

8. Carlier T, Eugène T, Bodet-Milin C, et al. Assessment of acquisition protocols for routine imaging of Y-90 using PET/CT. EJNMMI Res 2013;3:11.

9. Kao YH, Steinberg JD, Tay YS, et al. Post-radioembolization yttrium-90 PET/CT-part 1: diagnostic reporting. EJNMMI Res 2013;3:56.

10. Lea WB, Tapp KN, Tann M, et al. Microsphere localization and dose quantification using positron emission tomography/CT following hepatic intraarterial radioembolization with yttrium-90 in patients with advanced hepatocellular carcinoma. J Vasc Interv Radiol 2014;25:1595–603.

11. Pasciak AS, Bourgeois AC, Bradley YC. A comparison of techniques for ^{90}Y PET/CT image-based dosimetry following radioembolization with resin microspheres. Front Oncol 2014;4:121.

12. Attarwala AA, Molina-Duran F, Büsing KA, et al. Quantitative and qualitative assessment of yttrium-90 PET/CT imaging. PLoS One 2014;9:e110401.

13. Willowson KP, Tapner M, Bailey DL. A multicentre comparison of quantitative ^{90}Y PET/CT for dosimetric purposes after radioembolization with resin microspheres. Eur J Nucl Med Mol Imaging 2015; 42:1202–22.

14. D'Arienzo M, Pimpinella M, Capogni M, et al. Phantom validation of quantitative Y-90 PET/CT-based dosimetry in liver radioembolization. EJNMMI Res 2017;7:94.

15. Takahashi A, Himuro K, Baba S, et al. Comparison of TOF-PET and Bremsstrahlung SPECT images of yttrium-90: a Monte Carlo simulation study. Asia Ocean J Nucl Med Biol 2018;6:24.

16. Siman W, Mikell JK, Mawlawi OR, et al. Dose volume histogram-based optimization of image reconstruction parameters for quantitative ^{90}Y-PET imaging. Med Phys 2019;46(1):229–37.

17. Kao YH, Tan EH, Ng CE, et al. Yttrium-90 time-of-flight PET/CT is superior to Bremsstrahlung SPECT/CT for postradioembolization imaging of microsphere biodistribution. Clin Nucl Med 2011;36:186–7.

18. Kao YH, Tan EH, Lim KY, et al. Yttrium-90 internal pair production imaging using first generation PET/CT provides high-resolution images for qualitative diagnostic purposes. Br J Radiol 2012;85:1018–9.

19. Elschot M, Vermolen BJ, Lam MG, et al. Quantitative comparison of PET and Bremsstrahlung SPECT for imaging the in vivo yttrium-90 microsphere distribution after liver radioembolization. PLoS One 2013; 8(2):e55742.

20. Walrand S, Hesse S, Demonceau G, et al. Yttrium-90 labeled microspheres tracking during liver selective internal radiotherapy by bremsstrahlung pinhole SPECT: feasibility study and evaluation in an abdominal phantom. EJNMMI Res 2011;1:32.

21. Walrand S, Lhommel R, Goffette P, et al. Hemoglobin level significantly impacts the tumor cell survival fraction in humans after internal radiotherapy. EJNMMI Res 2012;2:20.

22. van den Hoven AF, Rosenbaum CE, Elias SG, et al. Insights into the dose-response relationship of radioembolization with resin ^{90}Y-microspheres: a prospective cohort study in patients with colorectal cancer liver metastases. J Nucl Med 2016;57:1014–9.

23. Chan KT, Alessio AM, Johnson GE, et al. Prospective trial using internal pair-production positron emission tomography to establish the yttrium-90 radioembolization dose required for response of hepatocellular carcinoma. Int J Radiat Oncol Biol Phys 2018;101:358–65.

24. Allimant C, Kafrouni M, Delicque J, et al. Tumor targeting and three-dimensional voxel-based dosimetry to predict tumor response, toxicity, and survival after yttrium-90 resin microsphere radioembolization in hepatocellular carcinoma. J Vasc Interv Radiol 2018;29:1662–70.

25. Ho CL, Chen S, Cheung SK, et al. Radioembolization with ^{90}Y glass microspheres for hepatocellular carcinoma: significance of pretreatment ^{11}C-acetate and ^{18}F-FDG PET/CT and posttreatment ^{90}Y PET/CT in individualized dose prescription. Eur J Nucl Med Mol Imaging 2018;45:2110–21.

26. Kennedy AS, Ball D, Cohen SJ, et al. Baseline hemoglobin and liver function predict tolerability and overall survival of patients receiving radioembolization for chemotherapy-refractory metastatic colorectal cancer. J Gastrointest Oncol 2017;8:70.

27. Strigari L, Sciuto R, Rea S, et al. Efficacy and toxicity related to treatment of hepatocellular carcinoma with ^{90}Y-SIR spheres: radiobiologic considerations. J Nucl Med 2010;51:1377–85.

28. Chiesa C, Mira M, Maccauro M, et al. Radioemboliza-tion of hepatocarcinoma with ^{90}Y glass microspheres: development of an individualized treatment planning strategy based on dosimetry and radiobiology. Eur J Nucl Med Mol Imaging 2015;42:1718–38.

29. Strydhorst J, Carlier T, Dieudonné A, et al. A gate evaluation of the sources of error in quantitative ^{90}Y PET. Med Phys 2016;43:5320–9.

30. Selwyn RG, Nickles RJ, Thomadsen BR, et al. A new internal pair production branching ratio of [90]Y: the development of a non-destructive assay for ^{90}Y and [90]Sr. Appl Radiat Isot 2007;65:318–27.

31. Rong X, Du Y, Ljungberg M, et al. Development and evaluation of an improved quantitative (90)Y brems-strahlung SPECT method. Med Phys 2012;39: 2346–58.

32. Conti M, Eriksson L. Physics of pure and non-pure positron emitters for PET: a review and a discussion. EJNMMI Phys 2016;3:8.

33. Walrand S, Jamar F, Mathieu I, et al. Quantitation in PET using isotopes emitting prompt single gammas: application to yttrium-86. Eur J Nucl Med Mol Imag-ing 2003;30:354–61.

34. Bagni O, D'Arienzo M, Chiaramida P, et al. ^{90}Y-PET for the assessment of microsphere biodistribution af-ter selective internal radiotherapy. Nucl Med Com-mun 2012;33:198–204.

35. Walrand S, Hesse M, Jamar F, et al. The origin and reduction of spurious extrahepatic counts observed in ^{90}Y non-TOF PET imaging post radioembolization. Phys Med Biol 2018;63:075016.

36. Cherry SR, Dahlbom M. Sensitivity: detector and geometric efficiencies. In: Phelps ME, editor. PET: physics, instrumentation and scanners. New York: Springer; 2008. p. 42–3.

37. Stabin MG, Sparks RB, Crowe E. OLINDA/EXM: the second-generation personal computer software for internal dose assessment in nuclear medicine. J Nucl Med 2005;46:1023–7.

38. Strother SC, Casey ME, Hoffman EJ. Measuring PET scanner sensitivity: relating countrates to image signal-to-noise ratios using noise equivalents counts. IEEE Trans Nucl Sci 1990;37:783–8.

39. Conti M. Effect of randoms on signal-to-noise ratio in TOF PET. IEEE Trans Nucl Sci 2006;53:1188–93.

40. Surti S, Kuhn A, Werner ME, et al. Performance of Philips Gemini TF PET/CT scanner with special consideration for its time-of-flight imaging capabil-ities. J Nucl Med 2007;48:471–80.

41. Walrand S, Hesse M, Chiesa C, et al. The low hepat-ic toxicity per Gray of ^{90}Y glass microspheres is linked to their transport in the arterial tree favoring a nonuniform trapping as observed in posttherapy PET imaging. J Nucl Med 2014;5:135–40.

42. Walrand S. Chapter 9. Microsphere deposition, dosimetry, radiobiology at the cell-scale, and predicted hepatic toxicity. In: Pasciak AS, McKinney JM, Bradley YC, editors. Handbook of ra-dioembolization, physics, biology, nuclear medicine, and imaging. Boca Raton (FL): CRC Press; 2016. Taylor & Francis.

43. Crookston NR, Fung GS, Frey EC. Development of a customizable hepatic arterial tree and particle trans-port model for use in treatment planning. IEEE Trans Radiat Plasma Med Sci 2018;3:31–7.

44. Högberg J, Rizell M, Hultborn R, et al. Heterogeneity of microsphere distribution in resected liver and tumour tissue following selective intrahepatic radio-therapy. EJNMMI Res 2014;4:48.

45. Högberg J, Rizell M, Hultborn R, et al. Increased ab-sorbed liver dose in Selective Internal Radiation Therapy (SIRT) correlates with increased sphere-cluster frequency and absorbed dose inhomogene-ity. EJNMMI Phys 2015;2:10.

46. Högberg J. Small-scale absorbed dose modelling in selective internal radiation therapy: microsphere dis-tribution in normal liver tissue. Gothenburg (MA): University of Gothenburg; 2015.

47. van de Maat GH, Seevinck PR, Elschot M, et al. MRI-based biodistribution assessment of holmium-166 poly(L-lactic acid) microspheres after radioemboli-sation. Eur Radiol 2013;23:827–35.

48. d'Abadie P, Hesse M, Jamar F, et al. [90]Y TOF-PET based EUD reunifies patient survival prediction in resin and glass microspheres radioembolization of HCC tumours. Phys Med Biol 2018;63:245010.

49. Chiesa C, Mira M, Maccauro M, et al. A dosimetric treatment planning strategy in radioembolization of hepatocarcinoma with ^{90}Y glass microspheres. Q J Nucl Med Mol Imaging 2012;56:503–8.

50. Mazzaferro V, Sposito C, Bhoori S, et al. Yttrium-90 radioembolization for intermediate-advanced hepa-tocellular carcinoma: a phase 2 study. Hepatology 2013;57:1826–37.

51. Kao YH, Steinberg JD, Tay Y-S, et al. Post-radioem-bolization yttrium-90 PET/CT part 2: dose-response and tumor predictive dosimetry for resin micro-spheres. EJNMMI Res 2013;3:57.

52. Bourgeois AC, Chang TT, Bradley YC, et al. Intra-procedural ^{90}Y PET/CT for treatment optimization of ^{90}Y radioembolization. J Vasc Interv Radiol 2014;25:271–5.

PET Assessment of Immune Effects from Interventional Oncology Procedures

Stephen J. Hunt, MD, PhD*, Siavash Mehdizadeh Seraj, MD, Abass Alavi, MD

KEYWORDS

- FDG-PET • Interventional oncology (IO) • Immunotherapy • Abscopal effect • Hyperprogression
- Pseudoprogression • iRECIST • Total lesion glycolysis (TLG)

KEY POINTS

- FDG-PET/CT has an expanding role in monitoring tumor response to immunotherapy.
- Interventional oncology procedures have the potential to alter tumor immune regulation.
- Complex patterns of immune response are reflected in complex patterns of imaging response in patients receiving both interventional oncology and immunotherapy.
- Morphologic measures of treatment response and immunologic response are inadequate and often inaccurate for measuring response in the setting of immune-mediated factors.
- FDG-PET has the potential to aid in both predicting and measuring immunologic treatment response.

INTRODUCTION

Interventional oncology (IO) locoregional therapies have become standard both as palliative and curative treatments in a variety of malignancies. Locoregional therapy (LRT) provides treatment options for patients with cancer not meeting criteria for curative resection; however, its efficacy is limited by tumor recurrence. By releasing tumor antigens and generating inflammation at the site of the tumor, however, multiple LRTs have shown potential for immune activation that could translate into improved efficacy and provide for systemic antitumor immunity.[1,2] Case reports of distant tumor regression in the setting of LRT demonstrate potential for immune-mediated regression, which are termed "abscopal" effects. The "acceleration" of the immune system provided by LRT, however, is generally insufficient for effective immune induction in the absence of immune coactivation or release of the "braking" mechanism of the regulatory immune system. The advent of new therapies for co-activating the immune system and inhibiting the regulatory immune mechanisms now opens the possibility for generating effective immune responses in combination with LRT.[1] LRT also has the potential to suppress antitumor immunity. To effectively examine these beneficial and untoward immune effects, however, quantitative measures of tumor response and immune activity are required.

FDG-PET imaging has become a prominent technique for diagnosis, staging, prognosis, and treatment response monitoring of different malignancies.[3] FDG-PET allows for quantification of tumor metabolism as measured by the magnitude of radiotracer uptake, which correlates with disease burden.[4] Activated immune cells, however, also

Disclosures: There are no relevant disclosures. Dr S.J. Hunt reports consulting and speaker fees unrelated to the study for Amgen, Inc. and BTG, PLC. Dr S.J. Hunt receives grant support from the NIH, Society of Interventional Radiology, American Cancer Society, and Society of Interventional Oncology.
Hospital of the University of Pennsylvania, Perelman School of Medicine, 3400 Spruce St., 1 Silverstein, Philadelphia, PA 19104, USA
* Corresponding author.
E-mail address: stephen.hunt@uphs.upenn.edu

PET Clin 14 (2019) 477–485
https://doi.org/10.1016/j.cpet.2019.06.007

demonstrate FDG uptake, which can obscure assessment of the true underlying disease burden and therapeutic efficacy.[5] Interventional oncologists must understand the underlying reasons for the disparate patterns of imaging responses due to underlying immune effects of LRT and immunotherapy. This review provides an overview of the immune effects of LRT, as well as the advantages and limitations of FDG-PET for tumor and immune response assessment.

THE TUMOR IMMUNE MICROENVIRONMENT

The immune system is a tightly regulated complex network that exists as a balance between immune activation and immune suppression. Too little immune induction, and the host is run over by infection and cancer. Too much immune induction, and autoimmunity develops. On the activation side, tumor cells express specific proteins and peptides called tumor-associated antigens (TAAs) that have the potential to activate the immune system.[6] These TAAs are presented on major histocompatibility I (MHC I) receptors in the tumor and are released from the cancer cell and internalized by antigen-presenting cells such as dendritic cells where they are presented on MHC II receptors. TAAs are then recognized by T helper cells (CD4+) and cytotoxic T lymphocytes (CTLs, CD8+) resulting in a forward feedback loop of immune activation, including cytokine release, activation of humoral immunity through B cells, complement and antibody production, and cell-mediated immunity through natural killer cell and CTL-mediated tumor killing.[7,8] These TAAs must be presented in the setting of additional costimulatory immune activation signals or they have the potential to induce tolerance to the antigen. Tolerance occurs through release of immunosuppressing cytokines that activate downstream immune regulatory cells resulting in immunosuppression. There are additional immune regulatory "checkpoints" consisting of specific cell surface receptors (eg, CTLA-4, PD-1) on regulatory T cells (Tregs) and myeloid derived suppressor cells and tumor cells (PDL1) that limit the magnitude of immune responses.[9] These checkpoints are often exploited by tumors to turn off the immune response. These suppressor cells infiltrate the tumor, and over time allow for its escape from immune-mediated tumor control.

EVIDENCE FOR LOCOREGIONAL THERAPY–INDUCED IMMUNE RESPONSE

The "abscopal effect" refers to the effect in which locoregional therapy of one site of cancer results in regression of distant "ab-scopus"; for example, "off-target" tumors. This effect was first described by Mole[10] in 1953 as an effect in radiation therapy whereby distant tumors occasionally regress in the setting of targeted radiation. Since that time, there have been at least 46 documented cases of the abscopal effect in radiation therapy.[11] A similar clinical effect has been described in other locoregional therapies, most notably cryoablation (CA), with additional indirect evidence of immune activation that does not result in sufficient activation for clinical tumor response.

Cryoablation

CA results in tumor destruction both through direct damage to tumor cell membranes and through thrombosis of tumor vasculature. CA is an attractive treatment modality from an immunologic perspective, as the mechanisms of action result in preservation of target immunogens and danger signals.[12] Preclinical studies have demonstrated immune induction by CA; however, there is also growing evidence of paradoxic immune inhibition in some settings.[12] This inhibition may be related to the induction of apoptosis instead of necrosis in slow-freeze versus fast-freeze methodology, with subsequent induction of the suppressor immune system.[13] In addition, immune activation appears to relate to the tumor volume, with larger tumor volumes possibly inducing anergy through the mechanism of high zone tolerance.[14] CA has the most robust clinical evidence of immune induction. Soanes and colleagues[15] provided the first clinical evidence of a systemic response to CA, noting regression of pulmonary and bone metastases in 2 patients with local CA of prostate cancer. Additional isolated cases of metastatic regression in prostate cancers treated with CA have been reported with subsequent palliation of bone pain.[16,17] Uhlschmid and colleagues[18] reported contralateral regression of lung tumors in 4 of 33 lung metastases treated with CA. Both Tanaka[19] and Suzuki[20] reported evidence from small case series of contralateral metastatic regression in patients with breast cancer treated with CA. Osada and colleagues[21] found evidence of distant tumor regression in 5 of 13 patients with liver metastases treated with CA, and in 1 of 3 patients with cholangiocarcinoma treated with CA. Most recently, Page and colleagues[22] presented evidence of induction of both humoral and cellular immunity in preoperative patients with breast cancer treated with a combination of CA and the CTLA-4 inhibitor, ipilimumab, with most patients treated with the combination therapy demonstrating an immune response in contrast to patients on either monotherapy alone.

Radiofrequency Ablation

Radiofrequency ablation (RFA) causes coagulative necrosis of tumors through a process of resistive heating caused by a high-frequency alternating current. The high temperatures generated (generally in the range of 60°–100°C) result in denaturing of protein content in the ablation zone; however, sublethal hyperthermia is notable at the tumor margin transitional zone. Numerous investigators have documented induction of heat shock proteins (HSPs) in the periablation zone and serum after RFA in both animals and humans.[23,24] These HSPs activate antigen-presenting dendritic cells, and elevated serum levels of HSP70 has been correlated with improved survival of patients treated with RFA.[3] Ali and colleagues[25] demonstrated a transient increase in activation of dendritic cells in the peripheral circulation of 5 patients with hepatocellular carcinoma (HCC) after RFA, resulting in their enhanced ability to stimulate CD4+ T cells. These patients also had increased serum levels of the proinflammatory cytokines tumor necrosis factor-α and interleukin (IL)-1β after RFA. There is little documented clinical evidence of abscopal effects in patients treated with RFA, and preclinical models suggest the CA is much more effective at inducing immune effects than RFA.[26–28]

Microwave Ablation

Microwave ablation (MWA) is a relatively newer modality for LRT that causes coagulative necrosis of tumors through hyperthermia induced by microwave energy deposition. Its primary clinical advantages are that it is faster, less susceptible to heat sink effects, and can treat larger tumors due to the synergistic effects of multiprobe activation. There are very few clinical reports of MWA-induced immune induction. Using pre-MWA and post-MWA biopsies, Zhang and colleagues[29] reported significant immune cell infiltration of HCC tumors after MWA in 82 patients, noting cell-type-specific time courses of infiltration after ablation. They also demonstrated immune infiltration of untreated HCC nodules in the opposite lobe after MWA, and reported a significant correlation between survival and the extent of immune infiltration. As in RFA, however, preclinical models suggest the immune-activating effects of MWA are far less than CA, possibly due to denaturing of the tumor antigens. For example, Ahmad and colleagues[30] demonstrated induction of HSP-70 and increases in IL-1β and IL-6 after MWA in a rat liver model; however, both immune effects were far more pronounced after CA in the same model.

High-Intensity Focused Ultrasound

High-intensity focused ultrasound (HIFU) exerts direct tumoricidal effects through frictional heating and mechanical cavitation and indirect effects through vascular thrombosis. Rosberger and colleagues[31] found an increase of the CD4+/CD8+ ratio in 3 of 5 patients receiving HIFU for choroidal melanoma. Other groups have since demonstrated similar differences in circulating T lymphocytes after HIFU in a variety of cancer subtypes including pancreatic cancer, osteosarcoma, HCC, and renal cell carcinoma.[32,33] Madersbacher and colleagues[34] demonstrated a significant induction of HSPs in prostate and bladder tumors treated with HIFU. They also demonstrated a significant increase in Th1-oriented tumor-infiltrating lymphocytes (TILs) and decrease in Th2-oriented (immunosuppressive) TILs in these patients.[35] Wu and colleagues[36] demonstrated similar findings of upregulation of HSPs and other danger signals in patients with breast cancer after HIFU with robust tumor infiltration of activated immune cells.[37,38]

Embolization

Transarterial embolization releases TAAs. Ayaru and colleagues[39] demonstrated an increase in the diversity and strength of TAA immune responses after embolization, an effect which is called "neo-antigenic expansion." Mizukoshi and colleagues[40] demonstrated that this "neo-antigenic expansion" after transarterial chemoembolization (TACE) can be amplified by blocking cytotoxic T-lymphocyte antigen-4 (CTLA-4) resulting in an unmasking of TAA-specific immune responses. Patients having TAA-specific T-cell responses after TACE have been demonstrated to have improved survival.[41] Liao and colleagues[42] reported that TACE increases circulating Th17 cells in a subset of patients with liver cancer, and this increase correlates with overall survival and time to progression. In addition, complex changes in inflammatory cytokine profiles after TACE, influence the immune response after therapy.[43]

IMAGING PATTERNS OF IMMUNE RESPONSE IN LOCOREGIONAL THERAPY

Morphologic cross-sectional measurements with or without contrast enhancement based on Response Evaluation Criteria In Solid Tumors (RECIST and mRECIST) represents the mainstay of imaging for assessing treatment response to locoregional therapy.[44] However, if we are to assume that LRTs can also have systemic effects, such as through hormonal signaling or immune induction, then a global assessment of systemic disease burden is needed to accurately stage a patient at baseline and determine a response in follow-up. Furthermore, one could expect that any systemic treatment response could be mixed, depending on the site of metastatic burden and underlying tumor heterogeneity. Although conventional PET measurements fail to capture the overall disease burden, quantitative measures of global disease metabolic activity can circumvent these challenges (**Fig. 1**).[45] Quantitative measures of global disease burden, including metabolic tumor volume, total lesion glycolysis (TLG), and partial volume–corrected total lesion glycolysis (pvcTLG) have been demonstrated to be predictive of treatment response and to be associated with survival outcomes in a wide variety of malignancies.[46–48] Finally, morphologic assessment of baseline disease burden using RECIST is not well correlated with treatment outcomes. On the other hand, baseline metabolic behavior has been demonstrated to predict disease response and to be correlated with molecular assessment of the tumor immune microenvironment, as measured by PD-1/PD-L1 positivity. For example, metabolic behavior of HCC at baseline as determined by fludeoxyglucose (FDG)-PET/computed tomography is superior to RECIST assessment for predicting survival outcome after Y90 radio-embolization.[49] In addition, FDG-PET uptake has been demonstrated to correlate with the expression of PD-1 and PD-L1 in bladder and lung cancer.[50,51] As these markers have been demonstrated to correlate patient treatment response, this suggests that pretreatment FDG-PET could serve as a biomarker for response to immunotherapy, the way microsatellite instability is used currently to stratify patients on their likelihood of therapeutic response.

Hyperprogression

In assessing response to any given therapy, one can imagine a number of different categories of response. In the worst case scenario, the therapy can induce growth of tumors distant from the treated lesion. This pattern of response has been dubbed "hyperprogression."[52] This effect is thought to be related either to stimulation of tumor growth due to inflammatory cytokine and hormone release caused by the treatment, or due to systemic immunosuppression caused by activation of the suppressive immune system (such as transforming growth factor-beta and IL-10 production) downstream of the inflammatory stimulus of the locoregional therapy.[53] Although anecdotally this effect is not uncommon in the setting of LRT, and the effect is quite common in preclinical models of LRT, unfortunately the interventional radiology literature is sparse in documenting the proportion of patients demonstrating hyperprogression.[54] This may in part relate to the difficulty in making quantitative assessments of global disease burden using morphologic measurement tools such as RECIST.

Pseudoprogression

Second, some proportion of patients may initially demonstrate apparent disease progression followed by treatment response. This pattern of response has been dubbed "pseudoprogression." Although most cases of apparent disease

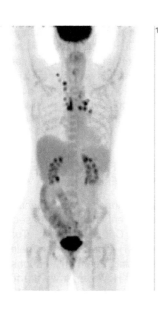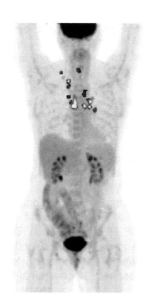

Fig. 1. Illustration of the workflow to quantify the global disease burden and treatment response in a patient with metastatic lung cancer. Pretreatment FDG-PET scan of a patient with metastatic lung cancer. The same PET images after segmentation of all active lesions using the adaptive thresholding system of ROVER software (ABX, Radeberg, Germany), which can extract quantitative PET parameters including total lesional glycolysis and partial volume–corrected total lesional glycolysis (TLG and pvcTLG). Subsequently, changes between baseline and follow-up imaging allow for assessment of overall response in the global burden of disease.

progression represent true progression, up to 15% of patients with melanoma on immunotherapy have been documented to experience pseudoprogression. This has led to modifying the standard RECIST criteria to incorporate "unconfirmed" progression requiring confirmation of progression on subsequent imaging (iRECIST), in particular for patients demonstrating clinical stability but progression on imaging.[55] As patients treated with LRT are increasingly receiving concomitant immunotherapy, it is important to be aware of this pattern of immune response, in particular in patients whose clinical condition appears to be improving in the setting of imaging suggestive of disease progression. Quantitative global disease burden assessment as reflected in TLG allows for accurate tracking of overall disease burden and pseudoprogression in the setting of heterogeneity of treatment response at any given tumor site (**Fig. 2**). Whether the combination of LRT and immunotherapy will demonstrate higher rates of pseudoprogression remains to be determined, but accurate assessment of global disease burden using quantitative measures of FDG-PET will allow for more accurate classification of patients into this pattern of response.

Abscopal Effects

Finally, some patients may indeed demonstrate distant tumor regression in the setting of locoregional therapy, aka, the "abscopal effect." Only a minority of patients will respond to checkpoint inhibitors, the most common type of immunotherapy. Theoretically, barriers to immunotherapy response can be overcome by combining the activating effects tumor antigen release with the inhibition of the regulatory immune populations with checkpoint inhibition.[1] In the setting of definite progression of disease on immunotherapy, the induction of a strong antitumor effect by a locoregional therapy has been definitively demonstrated in the setting of localized radiotherapy.[56] Twyman-Saint Victor and colleagues[56] demonstrated a larger proportion of major tumor regressions in a subset of patients with metastatic melanoma treated with the combination an anti-CTLA4 antibody (anti-CTLA4) and radiation. They proposed a mechanism whereby checkpoint inhibition promotes expansion of T cells, whereas radiation shapes the T-cell recepter repertoire of the expanded peripheral clones. Robust preclinical evidence suggests similar mechanisms for synergistic antitumor response in combination of immunotherapy and

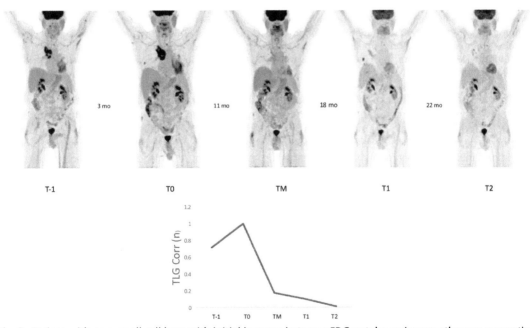

Fig. 2. Patient with non–small-cell lung with initial increase in tumor FDG uptake on immunotherapy, suggesting progression; however, later demonstrating sustained regression without addition of alternative therapy. At top, FDG-PET images illustrate the time course of treatment response demonstrating initial progression on immunotherapy followed by dramatic regression. This is the pattern of response dubbed "pseudoprogression," which can confound assessment of treatment response. At bottom, the quantitative global disease burden assessment as reflected in TLG using an adaptive contrast-oriented thresholding algorithm (ROVER software, ABX GmbH, Radeberg, Germany). (*Courtesy of* ROVER, ABX, Radberg, Germany.)

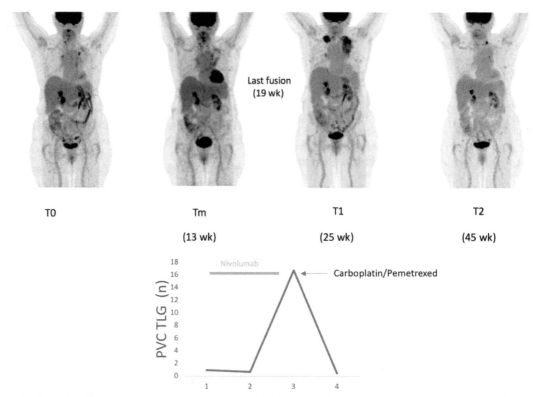

Fig. 3. Patient with non–small-cell lung cancer with initial stability followed by progression on immunotherapy, subsequently demonstrating a greater than expected robust response to salvage chemotherapy. At top, FDG-PET images illustrate the time course of treatment response demonstrating initial progression on immunotherapy followed by greater than expected dramatic regression after initiation of secondary therapy. This is the pattern of response expected if an LRT, such as ablation or embolization, initiates antitumor immunity (abscopal effect). At bottom, the quantitative global disease burden assessment, as reflected in pvcTLG, using an adaptive contrast-oriented thresholding algorithm (ROVER software, ABX GmbH, Radeberg, Germany). (*Courtesy of* ROVER, ABX, Radberg, Germany.)

LRT.[6,57,58] Isolated case reports of synergistic effects between LRT and immunotherapy also have been reported.[59,60] Multiple chemotherapies also have been demonstrated to reverse resistance to checkpoint inhibitors presumably through antigen exposure in the setting of chemotherapy-induced tumor cell death.[1] Again, quantitative global disease burden assessment as reflected in partial volume–corrected total lesion glycolysis (pvcTLG) allows for accurate tracking of overall disease burden and any reversal of immunotherapy resistance (**Fig. 3**). Whether the combination of LRT and immunotherapy will demonstrate higher rates of abscopal tumor responses remains to be determined, but accurate assessment of global disease burden using quantitative measures of FDG-PET will allow for more accurate classification of patients into this pattern of response.

Limitations

Any treatment effect that causes inflammation has the potential to obscure response assessment, as it becomes unclear whether hypermetabolic activity relates to tumor progression or uptake by the hypermetabolic immune cells. Indeed, pseudoprogression represents a specific example of this kind of limitation. There has been explosive growth in the past few years on the development of more specific radiotracers to differentiate progression from pseudoprogression and even characterize the different immune cell populations.[61]

SUMMARY

LRTs have the potential to induce immune responses that can be protumorigenic or antitumorigenic. Conventional measures of baseline disease and treatment response are insufficient to characterize the tumor immune microenvironment, to predict individual treatment responses, or to accurately assess the global burden of disease. Global disease measures of metabolic activity through FDG-PET have the potential to overcome some of these limitations. The rapid development of radiotracers that can differentiate between immune markers and populations will allow more precise targeting of immunotherapy and more robust predictions of tumor response.

REFERENCES

1. Chu KF, Dupuy DE. Thermal ablation of tumours: biological mechanisms and advances in therapy. Nat Rev Cancer 2014;14(3):199–208.

2. Mahajan A, Cook G. Clinical Applications of PET/CT in Oncology. In: Khalil M, editor. Basic Science of PET Imaging. New York: Springer Publishing; 2017. p. 429–50. https://doi.org/10.1007/978-3-319-40070-9_18.

3. Haen SP, Gouttefangeas C, Schmidt D, et al. Elevated serum levels of heat shock protein 70 can be detected after radiofrequency ablation. Cell Stress Chaperones 2011;16(5):495–504.

4. Basu S, Alavi A. PET-based personalized management in clinical oncology: an unavoidable path for the foreseeable future. PET Clin 2016. https://doi.org/10.1016/j.cpet.2016.03.002.

5. Aide N, Hicks RJ, Le Tourneau C, et al. FDG PET/CT for assessing tumour response to immunotherapy: report on the EANM symposium on immune modulation and recent review of the literature. Eur J Nucl Med Mol Imaging 2019. https://doi.org/10.1007/s00259-018-4171-4.

6. den Brok MHMGM, Sutmuller RPM, van der Voort R, et al. In situ tumor ablation creates an antigen source for the generation of antitumor immunity. Cancer Res 2004;64(11):4024–9.

7. Coulie PG, Hanagiri T, Takenoyama M. From tumor antigens to immunotherapy. Int J Clin Oncol 2001; 6(4):163–70.

8. Coulie PG, Van den Eynde BJ, van der Bruggen P, et al. Tumour antigens recognized by T lymphocytes: at the core of cancer immunotherapy. Nat Rev Cancer 2014;14(2):135–46.

9. Postow MA, Callahan MK, Wolchok JD. Immune checkpoint blockade in cancer therapy. J Clin Oncol 2015. https://doi.org/10.1200/JCO.2014.59.4358.

10. Mole RH. Whole body irradiation—radiobiology or medicine? Br J Radiol 1953. https://doi.org/10.1259/0007-1285-26-305-234.

11. Abuodeh Y, Venkat P, Kim S. Systematic review of case reports on the abscopal effect. Curr Probl Cancer 2016. https://doi.org/10.1016/j.currproblcancer.2015.10.001.

12. Sidana A. Cancer immunotherapy using tumor cryoablation. Immunotherapy 2014;6(1):85–93.

13. Sabel MS, Su G, Griffith KA, et al. Rate of freeze alters the immunologic response after cryoablation of breast cancer. Ann Surg Oncol 2010;17(4):1187–93.

14. Urano M, Tanaka C, Sugiyama Y, et al. Antitumor effects of residual tumor after cryoablation: the combined effect of residual tumor and a protein-bound polysaccharide on multiple liver metastases in a murine model. Cryobiology 2003;46(3):238–45.

15. Soanes WA, Ablin RJ, Gonder MJ. Remission of metastatic lesions following cryosurgery in prostatic cancer: immunologic considerations. J Urol 1970; 104(1):154–9.

16. Gursel E, Roberts M, Veenema RJ. Regression of prostatic cancer following sequential cryotherapy to the prostate. J Urol 1972;108(6):928–32.

17. Horan AH. Sequential cryotherapy for prostatic carcinoma: does it palliate the bone pain? Conn Med 1975;39(2):81–3.

18. Uhlschmid G, Kolb E, Largiader F. Cryosurgery of pulmonary metastases. Cryobiology 1979;16(2): 171–8.

19. Tanaka S. Cryosurgical treatment of advanced breast cancer. Skin Cancer 1995;10:9–18.

20. Suzuki Y. Cryosurgical treatment of advanced breast cancer and cryoimmunologic responses. Skin Cancer 1995;10(19–26).

21. Osada S, Imai H, Yawata K, et al. Growth inhibition of unresectable tumors induced by hepatic cryoablation: report of two cases. Hepatogastroenterology 2008;55(81):231–4.

22. Page DB, Ginsberg A, Dong Z, et al. Tumor and systemic immune responses to preoperative cryoablation plus immune therapy with ipilimumab in early-stage breast cancer. In: 2014 Breast Cancer Symposium. Vol 32. J Clin Oncol. 2014:[Abstract 64]. San Francisco, CA, September 4–6. 2014.

23. Schueller G, Kettenbach J, Sedivy R, et al. Heat shock protein expression induced by percutaneous radiofrequency ablation of hepatocellular carcinoma in vivo. Int J Oncol 2004;24(3):609–13.

24. Schueller G, Kettenbach J, Sedivy R, et al. Expression of heat shock proteins in human hepatocellular carcinoma after radiofrequency ablation in an animal model. Oncol Rep 2004;12(3):495–9.

25. Ali MY, Grimm CF, Ritter M, et al. Activation of dendritic cells by local ablation of hepatocellular carcinoma. J Hepatol 2005;43(5):817–22.

26. den Brok MHMGM, Sutmuller RPM, Nierkens S, et al. Efficient loading of dendritic cells following cryo and radiofrequency ablation in combination with immune modulation induces anti-tumour immunity. Br J Cancer 2006;95(7):896–905.

27. Jansen MC, van Hillegersberg R, Schoots IG, et al. Cryoablation induces greater inflammatory and coagulative responses than radiofrequency ablation or laser induced thermotherapy in a rat liver model. Surgery 2010;147(5):686–95.

28. Gao H-J, Zhang Y-J, Liang H-H, et al. Radiofrequency ablation does not induce the significant increase of CD4(+) CD25(+) Foxp3(+) regulatory T

cells compared with surgical resection in Hepal-6 tumor model. Arch Immunol Ther Exp (Warsz) 2013; 61(4):333–40.

29. Zhang J, Dong B, Liang P, et al. Significance of changes in local immunity in patients with hepatocellular carcinoma after percutaneous microwave coagulation therapy. Chin Med J (Engl) 2002; 115(9):1367–71.

30. Ahmad F, Gravante G, Bhardwaj N, et al. Changes in interleukin-1beta and 6 after hepatic microwave tissue ablation compared with radiofrequency, cryotherapy and surgical resections. Am J Surg 2010; 200(4):500–6.

31. Rosberger DF, Coleman DJ, Silverman R, et al. Immunomodulation in choroidal melanoma: reversal of inverted CD4/CD8 ratios following treatment with ultrasonic hyperthermia. Biotechnol Ther 1994;5(1–2):59–68.

32. Wang X, Sun J. High-intensity focused ultrasound in patients with late-stage pancreatic carcinoma. Chin Med J (Engl) 2002;115(9):1332–5.

33. Wu F, Wang Z-B, Lu P, et al. Activated anti-tumor immunity in cancer patients after high intensity focused ultrasound ablation. Ultrasound Med Biol 2004;30(9):1217–22.

34. Madersbacher S, Grobl M, Kramer G, et al. Regulation of heat shock protein 27 expression of prostatic cells in response to heat treatment. Prostate 1998; 37(3):174–81.

35. Kramer G, Steiner GE, Grobl M, et al. Response to sublethal heat treatment of prostatic tumor cells and of prostatic tumor infiltrating T-cells. Prostate 2004;58(2):109–20.

36. Wu F, Wang Z-B, Cao Y-D, et al. Expression of tumor antigens and heat-shock protein 70 in breast cancer cells after high-intensity focused ultrasound ablation. Ann Surg Oncol 2007;14(3):1237–42.

37. Lu P, Zhu X-Q, Xu Z-L, et al. Increased infiltration of activated tumor-infiltrating lymphocytes after high intensity focused ultrasound ablation of human breast cancer. Surgery 2009;145(3):286–93.

38. Xu Z-L, Zhu X-Q, Lu P, et al. Activation of tumor-infiltrating antigen presenting cells by high intensity focused ultrasound ablation of human breast cancer. Ultrasound Med Biol 2009;35(1):50–7.

39. Ayaru L, Pereira SP, Alisa A, et al. Unmasking of alpha-fetoprotein-specific CD4(+) T cell responses in hepatocellular carcinoma patients undergoing embolization. J Immunol 2007;178(3): 1914–22.

40. Mizukoshi E, Yamashita T, Arai K, et al. Enhancement of tumor-associated antigen-specific T cell responses by radiofrequency ablation of hepatocellular carcinoma. Hepatology 2013;57(4):1448–57.

41. Hiroishi K, Eguchi J, Baba T, et al. Strong CD8(+) T-cell responses against tumor-associated antigens prolong the recurrence-free interval after tumor treatment in patients with hepatocellular carcinoma. J Gastroenterol 2010;45(4):451–8.

42. Liao Y, Wang B, Huang ZL, et al. Increased circulating Th17 cells after transarterial chemoembolization correlate with improved survival in stage III hepatocellular carcinoma: a prospective study. PLoS One 2013. https://doi.org/10.1371/journal.pone.0060444.

43. Kim MJ, Jang JW, Oh BS, et al. Change in inflammatory cytokine profiles after transarterial chemotherapy in patients with hepatocellular carcinoma. Cytokine 2013. https://doi.org/10.1016/j.cyto.2013.07.021.

44. Therasse P, Arbuck SG, Eisenhauer EA, et al. New guidelines to evaluate the response to treatment. J Natl Cancer Inst 2000. https://doi.org/10.1093/jnci/92.3.205.

45. Torigian DA, Lopez RF, Alapati S, et al. Feasibility and performance of novel software to quantify metabolically active volumes and 3D partial volume corrected SUV and metabolic volumetric products of spinal bone marrow metastases on 18F-FDG-PET/CT. Hell J Nucl Med 2011;14(1):8–14.

46. Dholakia AS, Chaudhry M, Leal JP, et al. Baseline metabolic tumor volume and total lesion glycolysis are associated with survival outcomes in patients with locally advanced pancreatic cancer receiving stereotactic body radiation therapy. Int J Radiat Oncol Biol Phys 2014. https://doi.org/10.1016/j.ijrobp.2014.02.031.

47. Li Y-M, Lin Q, Zhao L, et al. Pre-treatment metabolic tumor volume and total lesion glycolysis are useful prognostic factors for esophageal squamous cell cancer patients. Asian Pac J Cancer Prev 2014. https://doi.org/10.7314/apjcp.2014.15.3.1369.

48. Lim R, Eaton A, Lee NY, et al. 18F-FDG PET/CT metabolic tumor volume and total lesion glycolysis predict outcome in oropharyngeal squamous cell carcinoma. J Nucl Med 2012. https://doi.org/10.2967/jnumed.111.101402.

49. Jreige M, Mitsakis P, Van Der Gucht A, et al. 18F-FDG PET/CT predicts survival after 90Y transarterial radioembolization in unresectable hepatocellular carcinoma. Eur J Nucl Med Mol Imaging 2017. https://doi.org/10.1007/s00259-017-3653-0.

50. Chen R, Zhou X, Liu J, et al. Relationship between the expression of PD-1/PD-L1 and 18 F-FDG uptake in bladder cancer. Eur J Nucl Med Mol Imaging 2019. https://doi.org/10.1007/s00259-018-4208-8.

51. Toschi L, Lopci E, Marchesi F, et al. A17Correlation of metabolic information on 18F-FDG PET with the tissue expression of immune markers in patients with non-small cell lung cancer (NSCLC) candidate to upfront surgery. Ann Oncol 2017. https://doi.org/10.1093/annonc/mdw332.17.

52. Champiat S, Ferrara R, Massard C, et al. Hyperprogressive disease: recognizing a novel pattern to improve patient management. Nat Rev Clin Oncol 2018. https://doi.org/10.1038/s41571-018-0111-2.

53. Fuentes-Antrás J, Provencio M, Díaz-Rubio E. Hyperprogression as a distinct outcome after immunotherapy. Cancer Treat Rev 2018. https://doi.org/10.1016/j.ctrv.2018.07.006.

54. Ahmed M, Kumar G, Moussa M, et al. Hepatic radiofrequency ablation–induced stimulation of distant tumor growth is suppressed by c-met inhibition. Radiology 2015. https://doi.org/10.1148/radiol.2015150080.

55. Seymour L, Bogaerts J, Perrone A, et al. iRECIST: guidelines for response criteria for use in trials testing immunotherapeutics. Lancet Oncol 2017. https://doi.org/10.1016/S1470-2045(17)30074-8.

56. Twyman-Saint Victor C, Rech AJ, Maity A, et al. Radiation and dual checkpoint blockade activate nonredundant immune mechanisms in cancer. Nature 2015. https://doi.org/10.1038/nature14292.

57. den Brok MHMGM, Sutmuller RPM, Nierkens S, et al. Synergy between in situ cryoablation and TLR9 stimulation results in a highly effective in vivo dendritic cell vaccine. Cancer Res 2006;66(14):7285–92.

58. Aarts BM, Klompenhouwer EG, Rice SL, et al. Cryoablation and immunotherapy: an overview of evidence on its synergy. Insights Imaging 2019;10(1):53.

59. Deipolyi AR, Bromberg JF, Erinjeri JP, et al. Abscopal effect after radioembolization for metastatic breast cancer in the setting of immunotherapy. J Vasc Interv Radiol 2018;29(3):432–3. https://doi.org/10.1016/j.jvir.2017.10.007.

60. Ghodadra A, Bhatt S, Camacho JC, et al. Abscopal effects and Yttrium-90 radioembolization. Cardiovasc Intervent Radiol 2016;39(7):1076–80. https://doi.org/10.1007/s00270-015-1259-0.

61. Solinas C, Porcu M, Hlavata Z, et al. Critical features and challenges associated with imaging in patients undergoing cancer immunotherapy. Crit Rev Oncol Hematol 2017;120:13–21.

Prostate-Specific Membrane Antigen PET/ Magnetic Resonance Imaging for the Planning of Salvage Radiotherapy in Patients with Prostate Cancer with Biochemical Recurrence After Radical Prostatectomy

Mattijs Elschot, PhD[a,b,*], Kirsten Margrete Selnæs, PhD[b],
Sverre Langørgen, MD[b], Håkon Johansen, MD[b],
Helena Bertilsson, MD, PhD[c,d], Torgrim Tandstad, MD, PhD[c,e],
Tone Frost Bathen, PhD[a,f]

KEYWORDS

- Prostate cancer • Recurrence • Prostatectomy • PSMA • PET • MR imaging
- Salvage radiotherapy

KEY POINTS

- Prostate-specific membrane antigen (PSMA) PET/magnetic resonance (MR) imaging can help distinguish between patients with prostate cancer with locoregional recurrence and those with distant metastases, even at low prostate-specific antigen levels.
- PSMA PET/MR imaging may have advantages compared with PET/computed tomography for the detection of local recurrence and anatomic correlates to PET-positive lymph node and bone lesions.
- PSMA PET/MR imaging can help in making informed treatment decisions in patients with biochemical recurrence after radical prostatectomy.
- PSMA PET/MR imaging enables dose-escalated and metastases-directed salvage radiotherapy in patients with biochemical recurrence after radical prostatectomy.

Disclosures: The researcher position of M. Elschot at the Norwegian University of Science and Technology is funded by the Central Norway Regional Health Authority. K.M. Selnæs, S. Langørgen, H. Johansen, H. Bertilsson, T. Tandstad, and T.F Bathen have nothing to disclose.

[a] Department of Circulation and Medical Imaging, Norwegian University of Science and Technology, PO Box 8900, NO-7491 Trondheim, Norway; [b] Department of Radiology and Nuclear Medicine, St. Olavs Hospital, Trondheim University Hospital, PO Box 3250 Torgarden, NO-7006 Trondheim, Norway; [c] Department of Cancer Research and Molecular Medicine, Norwegian University of Science and Technology, PO Box 8900, NO-7491 Trondheim, Norway; [d] Department of Urology, St. Olavs Hospital, Trondheim University Hospital, PO Box 3250 Torgarden, NO-7006 Trondheim, Norway; [e] The Cancer Clinic, St. Olavs Hospital, Trondheim University Hospital, PO Box 3250 Torgarden, NO-7006 Trondheim, Norway; [f] Department of Circulation and Medical Imaging. Norwegian University of Science and Technology, PO Box 8900, NO-7491 Trondheim, Norway
* Corresponding author. Department of Circulation and Medical Imaging, Norwegian University of Science and Technology, PO Box 8900, 7491 Trondheim, Norway.
E-mail address: mattijs.elschot@ntnu.no

PET Clin 14 (2019) 487–498
https://doi.org/10.1016/j.cpet.2019.06.003
1556-8598/19/© 2019 The Author(s). Published by Elsevier Inc. This is an open access article under the CC BY-NC-ND license (http://creativecommons.org/licenses/by-nc-nd/4.0/).

INTRODUCTION

Prostate cancer is the second most commonly diagnosed cancer type among men worldwide.[1] Over the last decades, the number of patients increased drastically because of increasing incidence and the wide availability of serum prostate-specific antigen (PSA) tests. Prostate cancer is a highly heterogeneous disease and patients are stratified in risk groups based on clinical factors such as PSA level, T stage, and Gleason grade.[2] Patients in the low-risk group usually do not require immediate treatment, but can be followed on active surveillance until disease progression warrants intervention. In contrast, patients in the intermediate-risk or high-risk group are usually offered radical treatment. Radical prostatectomy (RP) and radiotherapy (RT) are the 2 most common options for treatment with curative intent, with the former currently most used. However, approximately 30% of patients experience disease recurrence within 5 years after surgical removal of the prostate.[3,4]

Suspicion of prostate cancer recurrence is based on changes in PSA kinetics during the follow-up after initial treatment. After RP, biochemical recurrence (BCR) is defined as 2 consecutive increasing PSA values greater than 0.2 ng/mL.[5] To decide on treatment of recurrent disease, it is of utmost importance to distinguish between patients who have locoregional confined disease, which is considered curable, and those with distant metastases. Salvage radiotherapy (sRT) to the prostate bed and possibly pelvic lymph nodes, with or without short-term androgen deprivation therapy (ADT), is the standard treatment option for the first group, whereas palliative long-term ADT is the common treatment option for the latter.[5] However, patient stratification and treatment planning based on PSA values alone are challenging, because visual confirmation of the site of recurrence is lacking. Conventional imaging modalities are not sensitive enough to detect recurrent prostate cancer at the low PSA values with which patients typically present at the hospital.[5] Importantly, this caveat leads to a more or less blind treatment approach with associated risks of overtreatment of patients with occult metastatic disease, and suboptimal treatment of patients with potentially curable disease. An imaging examination that provides better knowledge of the site of recurrence would alleviate these problems and could enable more personalized treatment strategies.

Simultaneous PET/magnetic resonance (MR) imaging shows potential for improving the diagnosis in several cancer types.[6,7] For prostate cancer, PET/MR imaging with prostate-specific membrane antigen (PSMA) ligands can provide images with excellent soft tissue contrast, as well as a superior sensitivity for detection of recurrent disease.[8] This article discusses the emerging role of PSMA PET/MR imaging for the planning of sRT in patients with prostate cancer with BCR after RP.

SALVAGE RADIOTHERAPY AFTER RADICAL PROSTATECTOMY

sRT is defined as the administration of RT to the prostatic bed and possibly to the surrounding tissues, including lymph nodes, in patients with BCR after initial RP but no evidence of distant metastatic disease.[9] The main advantage of sRT compared with adjuvant RT (aRT), which is the administration of RT after RP but before evidence of disease recurrence, is that the former avoids overtreatment and associated side effects in patients who would never develop recurrent cancer.[9] One retrospective study with 510 patients found that the 8-year metastasis-free survival and overall survival did not differ significantly between pT3N0 patients receiving aRT (92% and 89%, respectively) or observation plus early sRT (91% and 92%, respectively).[10] Three ongoing prospective randomized controlled trials (ClinicalTrials.gov identifiers: NCT00541047, NCT00860652, NCT00667069) hope to shed more light on the potential differences in cancer control between aRT and sRT. Convincing evidence shows that sRT is most effective at low PSA values and should be commenced at the first signs of recurrence.[11–13] In a large multicenter study with patients initially treated with RP, Tendulkar and colleagues[13] reported 5-year absence of BCR in 71% of patients with pre-sRT PSA levels between 0.01 and 0.2 ng/mL, 63% for PSA 0.21 to 0.5 ng/mL, 54% for 0.51 to 1 ng/mL, 43% for 1.01 to 2 ng/mL, and 37% for PSA greater than 2 ng/mL. Likewise, the cumulative rate of distant metastases significantly correlated with pre-sRT PSA levels, ranging from 9% to 27% for the lowest and highest PSA groups, respectively. Results of the Radiation Therapy Oncology Group (RTOG) 9601 randomized controlled trial showed that the addition of 24 months of ADT to early sRT resulted in significantly higher rates for overall survival (76.3% vs 71.3%) and lower incidences of metastatic disease (14.5% vs 23%) and death from prostate cancer (5.8% vs 13.4%) at 12 years.[14] In the GETUG-AFU 16 randomized clinical trial, the addition of short-term ADT to early sRT had a significantly favorable effect on biochemical or clinical progression at 5-year follow-up (80% for sRT + ADT vs 62% for sRT alone), but no benefit on overall survival was found at time of analysis.[15] Similar results were recently reported from the interim analysis of the RTOG 0534 SPPORT trial, with 5-year freedom from progression in 71.1% of the patients who received prostate bed sRT alone versus 82.7% of patients who received sRT plus short-term ADT. A third arm with patients receiving additional irradiation of the pelvic lymph nodes showed significantly increased freedom from progression (89.1%) compared with the other 2 arms, as well as a significantly reduced likelihood of developing distant metastases at 8-year follow-up.[16] The reduced likelihood of developing distant metastases represents the first evidence from a randomized controlled trial that extending the sRT field to the pelvic lymph nodes leads to clinically meaningful reductions in BCR in patients without previous evidence of lymph node involvement (N0/Nx).

Computed tomography (CT) and bone scintigraphy (BS) are conventionally used to detect evidence of distant metastatic disease. However, these imaging modalities rarely detect disease at PSA levels less than 10 ng/mL, which limits their use for most candidates for sRT.[5] Consequently, patient selection for sRT and consecutive treatment planning is often based on PSA kinetics and other clinical parameters alone, without visual evidence of the site of recurrence. In general, a patient with prostate cancer with BCR after RP is considered a candidate for sRT if benefit from treatment may be expected, taking into consideration the risk of death unrelated to prostate cancer. The expected benefit of sRT is usually calculated using nomograms that typically include clinical parameters such as pre-sRT PSA, PSA doubling time, Gleason score, seminal vesicle invasion, extracapsular extension, surgical margins, lymph node metastases, concurrent or neoadjuvant ADT, and radiation dose to predict the risk of being progression free at some time after treatment.[11,13] In general, men with a life expectancy greater than 10 years may benefit from sRT, often given in combination with short-term ADT or antiandrogens (6–24 months). The total radiation dose given to the prostate bed should be at least 66 Gy.[5] A total radiation dose of 45 Gy to the whole pelvis is usually given in relapsing patients who had positive nodes on pelvic lymph node dissection (N1), although recent evidence shows that patients with negative or unknown pelvic lymph node stage (N0/Nx) may also benefit from pelvic lymph node irradiation.[16]

PROSTATE-SPECIFIC MEMBRANE ANTIGEN PET IMAGING

Clinical parameters are useful for predicting the patient's population-based probability of benefiting from sRT.[11,13] However, they do not provide direct evidence of the location of recurrence, which is of paramount importance for more tailored treatment. The ideal imaging examination would detect local recurrence in the prostate bed (T+), lymph node metastases inside (N1) and outside the pelvis (M1a), bone metastases (M1b) and other distant metastases (M1c) at low PSA levels, in order to facilitate informed clinical decision making based on the tumor-node-metastasis (TNM) staging system. However, traditional imaging modalities all have their limitations; CT is not useful for detection of local recurrence because of lack of soft tissue contrast, whereas both CT and BS lack sensitivity for detection of lymph node and bone metastases at low PSA levels.[17] MR imaging is excellent for assessment of local recurrence[18] but also performs poorly for detection of small lymph node metastases.[19]

Lately, there has been a strong focus on the development of prostate cancer–specific PET radiotracers, because alterations in molecular processes typically precede morphologic changes, thus providing opportunities for early detection of the site of recurrence. ^{11}C-choline and ^{18}F-fluciclovine are radiotracers that are currently US Food and Drug Administration approved for PET imaging in recurrent prostate cancer, whereas ^{18}F-fluoromethylcholine is often used in clinical practice as well. Most recently, PSMA-based radiotracers that are typically labeled with ^{68}Ga or ^{18}F, depending on the subtype, are rapidly gaining popularity for detection of recurrent prostate cancer. The current European Association of Urology (EAU) guidelines state that choline PET/CT may be useful in selected patients with PSA level greater than 1 ng/mL, especially when PSA doubling time is less than 6 months.[5] However, it has been consistently shown that choline PET has low detection rates at PSA levels less than 2 ng/mL.[20–22] In a head-to-head comparison in 100 patients with BCR after RP, fluciclovine PET showed higher detection rates than choline PET at PSA levels less than 2 ng/mL (21% vs 14% for PSA <1 ng/mL, 45% vs 29% for PSA 1–2 ng/mL).[23] Several studies compared PSMA PET with choline PET scans of the same patients, and higher detection rates were consistently found for the former, especially at PSA levels less than 1 ng/mL.[24–26] In a recent review of the available literature on these 3 radiotracers, Evans and colleagues[27] reported median PSMA PET detection rates of 51.5% for PSA level less than 1 ng/mL, 74% for PSA 1 to 2 ng/mL, and 90.5% for PSA greater than 2 ng/mL. These values compared favorably with those of choline PET (19.5% for PSA level <1 ng/mL, 44.5% for

PSA 1–2 ng/mL, and 76% for PSA >2 ng/mL) and fluciclovine PET (38% for PSA <1 ng/mL, 65% for PSA 1–2 ng/mL, and 78% for PSA >2 ng/mL). A large meta-analysis by Perera and colleagues[28] reported similar pooled detection rates for PSMA PET at low PSA levels. Specifically for patients with BCR after RP, these were 33% for PSA 0 to less than 0.2 ng/mL, 46% for PSA 0.2 to less than 0.5 ng/mL, 57% for PSA 0.5 to less than 1 ng/mL, 82% for PSA 1 to less than 2 ng/mL, and 97% for PSA greater than 2 ng/mL. Stratified by the site of recurrence, the pooled estimate of PSMA PET positivity for this patient group was 22% in the prostate bed, 36% in the pelvic lymph nodes, 7% in the extrapelvic lymph nodes, 15% in the bones, and 2% in the distant viscera.

In summary, PSMA ligands seem to outperform other prostate cancer–specific PET tracers, especially because of their ability to detect recurrent disease at PSA levels less than 1 ng/mL. Recurrence is more often detected outside than inside the prostate bed,[28] even at PSA levels less than 0.5 ng/mL,[29] which indicates that offering sRT to the prostate bed alone is suboptimal for most patients. One limitation is that reliable histologic verification of the PSMA PET findings is often lacking in the setting of recurrent prostate cancer. Although some studies have used biopsies to confirm subsets of PSMA PET-positive lesions, this approach does not provide information on lesions that are false-negative on imaging. Consequently, the best estimates of the sensitivity and specificity of PSMA PET in patients with BCR after RP are obtained from patients who have undergone dissection of the pelvic lymph nodes for primary staging. The pooled sensitivity and specificity of PSMA PET in this setting were shown to be 77% and 97%, respectively, on a per-patient analysis, and 75% and 99%, respectively, on a per-lesion analysis.[30]

PROSTATE-SPECIFIC MEMBRANE ANTIGEN PET/COMPUTED TOMOGRAPHY VERSUS PET/MAGNETIC RESONANCE IMAGING

Modern PET scanners are combined with a CT or MR imaging scanner to provide anatomic reference and morphologic correlates that are complementary to the molecular information from PET. To date, most PSMA PET studies have been performed on PET/CT scanners and some on PET/MR imaging scanners, reflecting the different availability of these scanners. Nevertheless, there may be advantages of using PET/MR imaging instead of PET/CT for detection of prostate cancer

recurrence, which can primarily be attributed to the superior soft tissue contrast of MR imaging compared with CT, as described later.

After RP and lymph node dissection, the anatomy of the pelvis is greatly changed. Multiparametric MR imaging (mpMR imaging), which is the combination of anatomic T2-weighted (T2w) MR images and functional dynamic contrast-enhanced (DCE) and diffusion-weighted (DW) MR images, allows differentiation between recurrent cancer, residual prostate tissue, inflammatory tissue, and fibrosis.[18] Although T2w MR imaging is mainly used for anatomic reference, the addition of DCE and, to some extent, DW MR imaging has been shown to significantly increase the sensitivity to detect locally recurrent disease.[31] Although the complementary nature of PSMA PET and MR imaging for detection of local recurrence remains to be clarified in large prospective studies, initial work with limited patient numbers and varying MR imaging protocols generally shows a favorable effect of combining the two modalities. In their study with 119 relapsing patients who underwent PSMA PET/CT and subsequent PET/MR imaging, Freitag and colleagues[32] found that mpMR imaging detected 18 cases of local recurrence, of which 9 were missed by the PET components of both PET/CT and PET/MR imaging. Lutje and colleagues[33] also detected more local recurrences with PET/MR imaging than with PET/CT (14 vs 9 in 25 patients), which was mainly attributed to the availability of MR images. In a small study with a trimodal PET/CT-MR imaging system, the addition of MR imaging was useful for cases with local recurrence, classified as indeterminate on PSMA PET/CT.[34] Lake and colleagues[35] found that DCE MR imaging was most effective for identifying PSMA-avid foci in the prostatic bed, and was able to detect additional lesions without associated PSMA uptake. The potential of PSMA PET/MR imaging for detection of local recurrence is further shown in **Fig. 1**, in which the mpMR imaging provides morphologic and functional correlates for a region with suspicious focal PSMA uptake in the prostate bed.

For detection of lymph node and bone metastases, superiority of PSMA PET compared with both MR imaging and CT has been clearly shown.[36–38] Nevertheless, PET/MR imaging may also have advantages compared with PET/CT in this setting. Freitag and colleagues[38] found that the visibility of the lymph nodes was significantly higher on MR imaging from PET/MR imaging compared with low-dose CT from PET/CT, as was the overall conspicuity for bone lesions. Similarly, Afshar-Oromieh and colleagues[39] stated that the different sequences and the higher resolution of MR

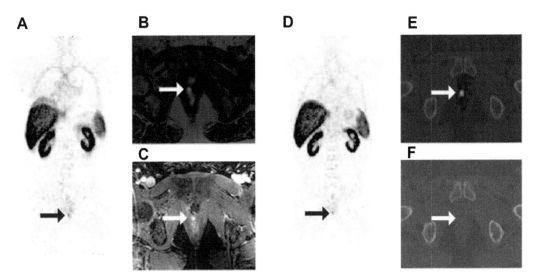

Fig. 1. PSMA-1007 PET/MR (*A–C*) and PET/CT (*D–F*) images of a patient with suspected local recurrence (*arrows*). Both PET from PET/MR imaging (*A*) and PET from PET/CT (*D*) show focal uptake in the prostate bed on the coronal images. PET image fusion with transverse T2w SPACE image provides soft tissue contrast for anatomic reference (*B*), whereas PET image fusion with the transverse low-dose CT image does not (*E*). Furthermore, early enhancement on the transverse DCE image provides another functional correlate (*C*), which is lacking on the low-dose CT image (*F*).

imaging enabled a subjectively easier evaluation of the PET/MR images compared with the PET/CT images. Lake and colleagues[35] reported that anatomic correlates were found on MR imaging for all suspected lymph node and bone metastases with focal PSMA PET uptake. These findings are supported by **Figs. 2** and **3**. They show that morphologic correlates to lymph node and bone lesions with focal PSMA uptake can be more easily identified on MR imaging than on low-dose CT.

The PET components of PET/CT and PET/MR imaging systems generally provide images of similar diagnostic quality, although standardized uptake values may differ because of differences in detector type and attenuation and scatter correction techniques.[40] Ringheim and colleagues[40] randomized the same-day scan order of PSMA PET/MR imaging and PET/CT and found that all suspected sites of local recurrence, lymph node, and bone metastases were visualized by both PET modalities. Similarly, Freitag and colleagues[38] found very high concordance for the detection of suspicious lymph nodes (98.5%) and bone metastases (100%) between PET from PET/MR imaging and PET from PET/CT. Of special concern are the photopenic (halo) artifacts around the bladder and kidneys that are sometimes present in PET images from PET/MR imaging but not from PET/CT.[38,39] These artifacts may especially hamper the evaluation of local recurrence and lymph node metastases in ^{68}Ga-PSMA-11 and ^{18}F-DCFPyl PET images, because these

PSMA variants are predominantly cleared by the kidneys. Halo artifacts are of less concern for ^{18}F-PSMA-1007, which has a predominant hepatic clearance.[41] Furthermore, it has been shown that, with simple adjustment of the maximum scatter fraction, these artifacts can be resolved.[42] One other concern with regard to PET/MR imaging is the long scan time, which may reduce its cost-effectiveness. Scan protocols may vary between PET/MR imaging scanners and PSMA ligands,[32,35,43] and international guidelines do not yet exist. In our institution, the total scan time of a whole-body ^{18}F-PMSA-1007 PET/MR imaging examination (4 bed positions, thighs to chin), including mpMR imaging of the prostate bed, is less than 45 minutes (**Table 1**). In clinical practice, this means that with PET/MR imaging 1 patient can be scanned every hour, whereas 2 patients per hour can be examined with PET/CT. In case of the latter, separate mpMR imaging of the prostate bed is also performed, usually in combination with MR imaging of the spine and the pelvic and abdominal lymph nodes, unless recent MR images are available. Consequently, the total scan time for PSMA PET/MR imaging is shorter than that of PMSA PET/CT plus MR imaging, with the additional advantage of intrinsically coregistered images.

The incorporation of MR imaging in RT target volume delineation has been shown to decrease the interobserver contouring variability compared with CT alone in patients with primary and

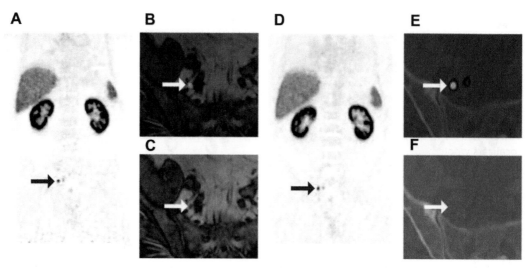

Fig. 2. PSMA-1007 PET/MR (*A–C*) and PET/CT (*D–F*) images of a patient with suspected lymph node metastases (*arrows*). Both PET from PET/MR imaging (*A*) and PET from PET/CT (*D*) show focal uptake in lymph nodes on the coronal images. PET image fusion with the transverse T1 weighted (T1w) volumetric interpolated breath-hold examination (VIBE) Dixon image provides soft tissue contrast for anatomic reference (*B*), whereas PET image fusion with the transverse low-dose CT image does not (*E*). Morphologic correlates to the suspected lymph nodes are more easily detected on the transverse T1w VIBE Dixon image (*C*) than on the transverse low-dose CT image (*F*).

recurrent prostate cancer.[44,45] However, MR imaging does not intrinsically provide information on the tissue's electron density for dose calculation and may suffer from geometric distortions, which traditionally limited its role as a stand-alone modality for RT planning. Now modern MR imaging hardware and software solutions have largely resolved these issues, MR imaging–only workflows are being implemented for RT of primary prostate cancer in clinical practice.[46] However, an MR imaging–only work flow would not be sufficient for dose-escalated and metastases-directed sRT in patients with prostate cancer with BCR after RP. Some investigators

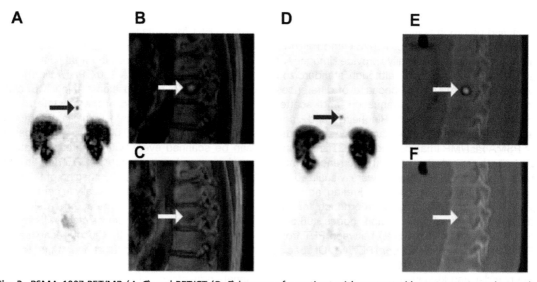

Fig. 3. PSMA-1007 PET/MR (*A–C*) and PET/CT (*D–F*) images of a patient with suspected bone metastases (*arrows*). Both PET from PET/MR imaging (*A*) and PET from PET/CT (*D*) show focal uptake in the spine on the coronal images. Both PET image fusion with the sagittal T1w turbo spin echo (TSE) image (*B*) and PET image fusion with the sagittal low-dose CT (*E*) provide anatomic reference in the bony tissue. However, the morphologic correlate to the suspected bone lesion may be more clearly visualized on the sagittal T1w TSE image than on the sagittal low-dose CT image (*F*).

Table 1
The PET/magnetic resonance imaging scan protocol and corresponding scan times (minutes) used on the 3-T Biograph mMR scanner (Siemens Healthineers, Erlangen, Germany) in our institution

MR Imaging Sequence	Simultaneous PET
Localizers whole body (2:45)	No
4 bed positions MRAC (0:15) T1w VIBE COR (0:15) T2w HASTE TRA (1:15) DW EPI TRA (2:28) T1w TSE SAG (0:58)	Yes (6:00)
Localizer pelvis (0:57)	No
1 bed position MRAC (0:15) T2w SPACE (08:15)	Yes (10:00)
DW EPI TRA (3:33)	No
DCE T1w VIBE TRA (3:29)	No

In patients who have undergone prostatectomy, typical high-resolution T2w turbo spin echo imaging of the prostate bed in 3 orthogonal planes is deemed unnecessary when high-resolution (0.5 × 0.5 × 1 mm³) T2w SPACE images are also available.

Abbreviations: COR, coronal; DW EPI, Diffusion-weighted echo planar imaging; HASTE, half-Fourier acquired single-shot turbo spin echo; MRAC, MR imaging–based attenuation correction; SAG, sagittal; SPACE, Sampling Perfection with Application optimized Contrasts using different flip angle Evolution; T1w, T1 weighted; TRA, transverse; TSE, turbo spin echo; VIBE, volumetric interpolated breath-hold examination.

have suggested a PSMA PET/CT-based workflow,[47,48] but this approach would still suffer from the inherent limitations of CT. For example, Habl and colleagues[49] reported that additional planning MR imaging needed to be performed when PSMA PET/CT suggested local recurrence, because morphologic correlates were usually lacking in the CT scan. In contrast, a PSMA PET/MR imaging–based RT planning workflow could provide all the information needed for delineation of the target volumes and organs at risk.

IMPACT OF PROSTATE-SPECIFIC MEMBRANE ANTIGEN PET ON PATIENT MANAGEMENT

According to international guidelines,[5] patients with BCR after RP should be treated with sRT when PSA levels are less than 0.5 ng/mL, presuming the site of recurrence is locally in the prostate bed. It has been shown that the therapeutic effect of sRT reduces with increasing PSA levels,[12,13] which probably reflects an increased likelihood of occult metastatic disease outside the radiation field. However, even in the low-PSA group, more than 40% of patients treated with sRT do not achieve long-term PSA response.[50] New insights into the pattern of prostate cancer recurrence came to light with the introduction of PSMA PET imaging, among other things convincingly showing that low PSA values do not guarantee absence of metastatic disease.[29,47] For example, one study by Meredith and colleagues[29] reported suspected local recurrence, lymph node metastases, and bone metastases in 2%, 7%, and 2% of patients with PSA level less than 0.2 ng/mL, respectively, and in 8%, 13%, and 6% of patients with PSA 0.2 to less than 0.5 ng/mL. This pattern of recurrence at low PSA values mimics more or less the overall pattern described in the meta-analysis by Perera and colleagues,[28] albeit with lower detection rates. Consequently, PSMA PET imaging may be the key to improving the efficacy of sRT, by unblinding the patient selection and treatment planning process, and a substantial impact on patient management may be expected.

A recent meta-analysis by Han and colleagues[51] showed that PSMA PET imaging changed treatment decisions in about half of all patients with prostate cancer. They pooled the results obtained from studies with a mix of patients with prostate cancer, including those with primary prostate cancer, BCR after RP, and BCR after RT, and found an overall proportion of (intended or implemented) change in management of 54%. PET positivity was the only variable significantly associated with a change in management. In patients with BCR after initial treatment (RP, RT, or both), the availability of PSMA PET led to increased use of curative treatment options at the expense of palliative systemic treatment. The proportion of patients assigned to radiotherapy increased from 56% before PSMA PET to 62% after PSMA PET, surgery increased from 1% to 7%, focal treatment from 1% to 2%, and multimodal treatment from 2% to 6%. In contrast, the proportion of patients assigned to systemic treatment decreased from 26% to 12% because of PSMA PET, and those without treatment decision decreased from 14% to 11%. Conventional sRT to the prostate bed was the RT methodology of choice in 95% of the patients before PSMA PET imaging. However, after PSMA PET, 24% of patients received sRT with increased dose to the sites of suspected recurrence and/or an enlarged target volume, including the sites of recurrence, and 20% received stereotactic body RT to single metastases or oligometastases. There was a tendency toward a greater proportion of change in patient management in studies that included relapsing patients with higher PSA levels (43% for PSA <1 ng/mL, 54% for PSA 1 to <2 ng/mL, and 69% for PSA >2 ng/mL).

For this work, 10 studies that specifically reported the overall change in management in patients with BCR after RP were identified (Table 2). Major changes in treatment management were reported in 19% to 77% of patients, with a 43% median proportion of change. This finding agrees well with the pooled proportion of change for the lowest PSA level group (<1 ng/mL) reported by Han and colleagues,[51] which is based on patients initially treated with RP (±RT) only.[49,52,53] Seven out of 10 studies explicitly reported the changes in treatment decisions.[47–49,52–55] Van Leeuwen and colleagues[53] investigated the impact of PMSA PET in men who were diagnosed with BCR after RP and were being considered for sRT to the prostate bed. PSMA PET changed the treatment in 20 out of 70 (29%) patients, including enlarging the RT treatment volume to the pelvic nodes in 5 out of 20 (25%) patients, changing to surgical salvage lymph node dissection in 1 out of 20 (5%) patients, RT to the pelvic lymph nodes plus ADT in 6 out of 20 (30%) patients, stereotactic RT of a solitary pelvic lymph node in 4 out of 20 (20%) patients, stereotactic RT of a lesion outside the pelvis with or without ADT in 3 out of 20 (15%) patients, and RT to the prostatic fossa plus stereotactic radiotherapy for an extrapelvic lesion in 1 out of 20 (5%) patients. Bluemel and colleagues[54] investigated the impact of PSMA PET on patient management in men with persistent PSA or BCR after RP and who were candidates for sRT to the prostate bed. Treatment recommendations changed in 19 out of 42 (42%) patients because

of findings on PSMA PET. These changes included dose escalation to local recurrence in 6 out of 19 patients (32%); extension of the RT field to a suspicious rectal lesion in 2 out of 19 (11%) patients; extension of the RT field to pelvic and/or retroperitoneal lymph node metastases, including dose escalation for involved lymph nodes in 8 out of 19 (42%) patients; extension of the RT field to lymph node metastases and a single bone metastasis in 1 out of 19 (5%) patients; and change to systemic treatment with ADT in 2 out of 19 (11%) patients with multiple distant bone metastases and/or multiple lymph node metastases. Habl and colleagues[49] investigated the impact of PSMA PET on sRT treatment planning in 100 patients with BCR after RP, with or without prior RT. Only patients who received sRT after PSMA PET imaging were considered, thus, for example, excluding patients with multiple metastases who received ADT or other therapies. The conventional RT treatment plan (prostate bed) was changed in 59 out of 100 (59%) patients. These plans included RT plus simultaneous integrated boost (SIB) to the prostate bed in 19 out of 59 (32%) patients, RT plus SIB to the pelvic lymph nodes in 22 out of 59 (37%) patients, RT plus SIB to extrapelvic lymph nodes in 15 out of 59 (25%) patients, stereotactic RT to a single lymph node metastasis in 1 out of 59 (2%) patients, and stereotactic RT bone metastases in 10 out of 59 (17%) patients. Zschaek and colleagues[55] investigated the impact of PSMA PET on treatment management in high-risk patients presenting with BCR after RP and who were candidates for sRT. All 22 patients were originally scheduled for sRT of the prostate bed. PSMA PET led to treatment modifications in 17 out of 22 (77%) patients, including an additional

Table 2
Overview of studies that report the impact of prostate-specific membrane antigen PET on treatment decisions, specifically for patients with prostate cancer with biochemical recurrence after radical prostatectomy

Study by First Author	N	Average Age (y)	Average PSA (ng/mL)	Detection Rate (%)	Proportion of Change in Management (%)
Sterzing et al,[56] 2016	42	70	2.8	74	61
Van Leeuwen et al,[53] 2016	70	67	0.2	54	29
Bluemel et al,[54] 2016	46	69	0.7	53	42
Habl et al,[49] 2017	100	64	0.7	71	59
Hope et al,[57] 2017	43	69	2.7	—	33
Afaq et al,[58] 2018	68	—	—	—	34
Zschaeck et al,[55] 2017	22	65	6.1	—	77
Grubmüller et al,[52] 2018	117	74	1.0	86	43
Henkenberens et al,[48] 2018	39	66	1.2	85	59
Calais et al,[47] 2018	270	68	0.4	49	19

dose boost to local recurrence in 6 out of 17 (35%) patients, extension of the RT field plus an additional dose boost to the affected lymph nodes in 10 out of 17 (59%) patients, and stereotactic RT of bone metastases in 4 out of 17 (24%) patients. In 1 out of 17 (6%) patients, RT was omitted because of extensive metastatic disease. Grubmuller and colleagues[52] found that PSMA PET changed the clinical decision-making in 50 out of 117 (42%) patients with BCR after RP, with or without prior RT. RT to the prostate bed was changed to wait and see in 1 out of 50 (2%) patients, to salvage surgery in 1 out of 50 (2%) patients, and to metastases-directed RT in 1 out of 50 (2%) patients. ADT was changed to wait and see in 1 out of 50 (2%) patients, to salvage surgery in 10 out of 50 (20%) patients, to metastases-directed RT in 13 out of 50 (26%) patients, and to multimodal treatment in 5 out of 50 (10%) patients. Wait and see was changed to salvage surgery in 2 out of 50 (4%) patients and to metastases-directed RT in 16 out of 50 (32%) patients. Henkenberens and colleagues[48] also investigated the impact of PSMA PET on the management of relapsing patients with a high risk of metastatic disease. Treatment was changed from conventional sRT to the prostate bed to individualized treatment concepts in 23 out of 39 (59%) patients, including metastases-directed RT with or without ADT in 19 out of 23 (83%) patients, ADT alone in 2 out of 23 (9%) patients, chemotherapy alone in 1 out of 23 (4%) patients, and ADT plus chemotherapy in 1 out of 23 (4%) patients. In addition, Calais and colleagues[47] investigated the potential impact of PSMA PET on the planning of sRT in patients with PSA levels less than 1 ng/mL. Major impact was found in 52 out of 270 (19%) patients, including extension of the pelvic target volume in 19 out of 52 (37%) patients, extension of the target volume to the para-aortic lymph nodes in 5 out of 52 (10%) patients, and metastases-directed stereotactic body RT in 22 out of 52 (42%) patients. In 6 out of 52 (12%) patients, RT would have been avoided because of advanced metastatic disease. In addition, 80 out of 270 (30%) patients could have received focal dose escalation to lesions within the original target volume, which was considered as minor impact by the investigators.

In summary, these initial studies indicate that PSMA PET can have substantial impact on the planning of sRT in patients with prostate cancer with BCR after RP. Some patients received palliative systemic treatment because PSMA PET indicated that sRT would be futile because of the presence of advanced metastatic disease. In other patients, long-term ADT was modified to locoregional sRT, thereby potentially curing the disease and reducing, or at least delaying, systemic side effects. In a substantial number of patients, the RT plan was adapted to include all sites of recurrence, to boost the dose to suspected lesions, and/or to treat single or oligometastatic disease. In others, PSMA PET revealed that active treatment and not a wait-and-see policy would be the best treatment strategy to avoid progression of existing disease. Importantly, these findings cannot be generalized to all relapsing patients after RP because of limitations with regard to retrospective study design, low numbers of patients, mixed populations, and patient selection bias. Furthermore, long-term follow-up data are currently lacking, so it remains to be seen whether PSMA PET-based treatment planning will lead to improved overall survival. Two prospective randomized controlled trials (ClinicalTrials.gov identifier: NCT03525288, NCT03582774) are currently underway to shed more light on these important questions.

SUMMARY

sRT is a potentially curative treatment option for patients with prostate cancer with BCR after RP, especially when PSA levels are still low. Because of a lack of sensitive conventional imaging methods, the planning of sRT is currently being performed in the absence of visual evidence of the site of recurrence. Simultaneous PSMA PET/MR imaging combines excellent soft tissue contrast with a superior sensitivity for cancer, and can help detect recurrence in the prostate bed, lymph nodes, bones, and distant organs. Consequently, PSMA PET/MR imaging can play an important role in the selection of patients who may benefit from sRT, and facilitate dose-escalated and metastases-directed treatment planning. Whether or not PSMA PET/MR imaging–based planning of sRT can improve the long-term outcome in patients with BCR after RP should be answered in prospective randomized controlled trials.

REFERENCES

1. Siegel RL, Miller KD, Jemal A. Cancer statistics, 2017. CA Cancer J Clin 2017;67(1):7–30.
2. Mottet N, Bellmunt J, Bolla M, et al. EAU-ESTRO-SIOG Guidelines on prostate cancer. Part 1: screening, diagnosis, and local treatment with curative intent. Eur Urol 2017;71(4):618–29.
3. Freedland SJ, Presti JC, Amling CL, et al. Time trends in biochemical recurrence after radical prostatectomy: results of the SEARCH database. Urology 2003; 61(4):736–41. Available at: http://www.ncbi.nlm.nih.

gov/pubmed/12670557. Accessed February 28, 2019.

4. Ward JF, Blute ML, Slezak J, et al. The Long-term clinical impact of biochemical recurrence of prostate cancer 5 or more years after radical prostatectomy. J Urol 2003;170(5):1872–6.

5. Cornford P, Bellmunt J, Bolla M, et al. EAU-ESTRO-SIOG guidelines on prostate cancer. Part II: treatment of relapsing, metastatic, and castration-resistant prostate cancer. Eur Urol 2017;71(4):630–42.

6. Sotoudeh H, Sharma A, Fowler KJ, et al. Clinical application of PET/MRI in oncology. J Magn Reson Imaging 2016;44(2):265–76.

7. Kwon HW, Becker A-K, Goo JM, et al. FDG whole-body PET/MRI in oncology: a systematic review. Nucl Med Mol Imaging 2017;51(1):22–31.

8. Barbosa F, Queiroz M, Nunes R, et al. Clinical perspectives of PSMA PET/MRI for prostate cancer. Clinics 2018;73(Suppl 1).

9. Thompson IM, Valicenti RK, Albertsen P, et al. Adjuvant and salvage radiotherapy after prostatectomy: AUA/ASTRO Guideline. J Urol 2013;190(2):441–9.

10. Fossati N, Karnes RJ, Boorjian SA, et al. Long-term impact of adjuvant versus early salvage radiation therapy in pT3N0 prostate cancer patients treated with radical prostatectomy: results from a multi-institutional series. Eur Urol 2017;71(6):886–93.

11. Stephenson AJ, Scardino PT, Kattan MW, et al. Predicting the outcome of salvage radiation therapy for recurrent prostate cancer after radical prostatectomy. J Clin Oncol 2007;25(15):2035–41.

12. Pfister D, Bolla M, Briganti A, et al. Early salvage radiotherapy following radical prostatectomy. Eur Urol 2014;65(6):1034–43.

13. Tendulkar RD, Agrawal S, Gao T, et al. Contemporary update of a multi-institutional predictive nomogram for salvage radiotherapy after radical prostatectomy. J Clin Oncol 2016;34(30):3648–54.

14. Shipley WU, Seiferheld W, Lukka HR, et al. Radiation with or without antiandrogen therapy in recurrent prostate cancer. N Engl J Med 2017;376(5):417–28.

15. Carrie C, Hasbini A, de Laroche G, et al. Salvage radiotherapy with or without short-term hormone therapy for rising prostate-specific antigen concentration after radical prostatectomy (GETUG-AFU 16): a randomised, multicentre, open-label phase 3 trial. Lancet Oncol 2016;17(6):747–56.

16. Pollack A, Karrison TG, Balogh AG, et al. Short term androgen deprivation therapy without or with pelvic lymph node treatment added to prostate bed only salvage radiotherapy: the NRG oncology/RTOG 0534 SPPORT trial. Int J Radiat Oncol 2018;102(5):1605.

17. Kane CJ, Amling CL, Johnstone PA, et al. Limited value of bone scintigraphy and computed tomography in assessing biochemical failure after radical prostatectomy. Urology 2003;61(3):607–11.

18. Gaur S, Turkbey B. Prostate MR imaging for post-treatment evaluation and recurrence. Radiol Clin North Am 2018;56(2):263–75.

19. Hövels AM, Heesakkers RAM, Adang EM, et al. The diagnostic accuracy of CT and MRI in the staging of pelvic lymph nodes in patients with prostate cancer: a meta-analysis. Clin Radiol 2008;63(4):387–95.

20. Krause BJ, Souvatzoglou M, Tuncel M, et al. The detection rate of [11C]Choline-PET/CT depends on the serum PSA-value in patients with biochemical recurrence of prostate cancer. Eur J Nucl Med Mol Imaging 2008;35(1):18–23.

21. Castellucci P, Ceci F, Graziani T, et al. Early biochemical relapse after radical prostatectomy: which prostate cancer patients may benefit from a restaging 11C-Choline PET/CT scan before salvage radiation therapy? J Nucl Med 2014;55(9):1424–9.

22. Giovacchini G, Picchio M, Briganti A, et al. [^{11}C] Choline positron emission tomography/computerized tomography to restage prostate cancer cases with biochemical failure after radical prostatectomy and no disease evidence on conventional imaging. J Urol 2010;184(3):938–43. https://doi.org/10.1016/j.juro.2010.04.084.

23. Nanni C, Zanoni L, Pultrone C, et al. 18F-FACBC (anti1-amino-3-18F-fluorocyclobutane-1-carboxylic acid) versus 11C-choline PET/CT in prostate cancer relapse: results of a prospective trial. Eur J Nucl Med Mol Imaging 2016;43(9):1601–10.

24. Morigi JJ, Stricker PD, van Leeuwen PJ, et al. Prospective comparison of 18F-Fluoromethylcholine versus 68Ga-PSMA PET/CT in prostate cancer patients who have rising PSA after curative treatment and are being considered for targeted therapy. J Nucl Med 2015;56(8):1185–90.

25. Afshar-Oromieh A, Zechmann CM, Malcher A, et al. Comparison of PET imaging with a 68Ga-labelled PSMA ligand and 18F-choline-based PET/CT for the diagnosis of recurrent prostate cancer. Eur J Nucl Med Mol Imaging 2014;41(1):11–20.

26. Schwenck J, Rempp H, Reischl G, et al. Comparison of 68Ga-labelled PSMA-11 and 11C-choline in the detection of prostate cancer metastases by PET/CT. Eur J Nucl Med Mol Imaging 2017;44(1):92–101.

27. Evans JD, Jethwa KR, Ost P, et al. Prostate cancer–specific PET radiotracers: a review on the clinical utility in recurrent disease. Pract Radiat Oncol 2018;8(1):28–39.

28. Perera M, Papa N, Roberts M, et al. Gallium-68 prostate-specific membrane antigen positron emission tomography in advanced prostate cancer—updated diagnostic utility, sensitivity, specificity, and distribution of prostate-specific membrane antigen-avid lesions: a systematic review and meta-analysis. Eur Urol 2019. https://doi.org/10.1016/J.EURURO.2019.01.049.

29. Meredith G, Wong D, Yaxley J, et al. The use of [68] Ga-PSMA PET CT in men with biochemical recurrence after definitive treatment of acinar prostate cancer. BJU Int 2016;118:49–55.

30. Perera M, Papa N, Christidis D, et al. Sensitivity, specificity, and predictors of positive 68 Ga–prostate-specific membrane antigen positron emission tomography in advanced prostate cancer: a systematic review and meta-analysis. Eur Urol 2016;70(6):926–37.

31. Panebianco V, Barchetti F, Sciarra A, et al. Prostate cancer recurrence after radical prostatectomy: the role of 3-T diffusion imaging in multi-parametric magnetic resonance imaging. Eur Radiol 2013; 23(6):1745–52.

32. Freitag MT, Radtke JP, Afshar-Oromieh A, et al. Local recurrence of prostate cancer after radical prostatectomy is at risk to be missed in 68Ga-PSMA-11-PET of PET/CT and PET/MRI: comparison with mpMRI integrated in simultaneous PET/MRI. Eur J Nucl Med Mol Imaging 2017;44(5):776–87.

33. Lütje S, Cohnen J, Gomez B, et al. Integrated 68Ga-HBED-CC-PSMAPET/MRI in patients with suspected recurrent prostate cancer. Nuklearmedizin 2017; 56(03):73–81.

34. Alonso O, dos Santos G, García Fontes M, et al. 68Ga-PSMA and 11C-Choline comparison using a tri-modality PET/CT-MRI (3.0 T) system with a dedicated shuttle. Eur J Hybrid Imaging 2018;2(1):9.

35. Lake ST, Greene KL, Westphalen AC, et al. Optimal MRI sequences for 68Ga-PSMA-11 PET/MRI in evaluation of biochemically recurrent prostate cancer. EJNMMI Res 2017;7(1):77.

36. Dyrberg E, Hendel HW, Huynh THV, et al. 68Ga-PSMA-PET/CT in comparison with 18F-fluoride-PET/CT and whole-body MRI for the detection of bone metastases in patients with prostate cancer: a prospective diagnostic accuracy study. Eur Radiol 2019;29(3):1221–30.

37. Zacho HD, Nielsen JB, Afshar-Oromieh A, et al. Prospective comparison of 68Ga-PSMA PET/CT, 18F-sodium fluoride PET/CT and diffusion weighted-MRI at for the detection of bone metastases in biochemically recurrent prostate cancer. Eur J Nucl Med Mol Imaging 2018;45(11):1884–97.

38. Freitag MT, Radtke JP, Hadaschik BA, et al. Comparison of hybrid 68Ga-PSMA PET/MRI and 68Ga-PSMA PET/CT in the evaluation of lymph node and bone metastases of prostate cancer. Eur J Nucl Med Mol Imaging 2016;43(1):70–83.

39. Afshar-Oromieh A, Haberkorn U, Schlemmer HP, et al. Comparison of PET/CT and PET/MRI hybrid systems using a 68Ga-labelled PSMA ligand for the diagnosis of recurrent prostate cancer: initial experience. Eur J Nucl Med Mol Imaging 2014; 41(5):887–97.

40. Ringheim A, Campos Neto GC, Martins KM, et al. Reproducibility of standardized uptake values of same-day randomized 68Ga-PSMA-11 PET/CT and PET/MR scans in recurrent prostate cancer patients. Ann Nucl Med 2018;32(8):523–31.

41. Giesel FL, Will L, Lawal I, et al. Intraindividual comparison of [18] F-PSMA-1007 and [18] F-DCFPyL PET/CT in the prospective evaluation of patients with newly diagnosed prostate carcinoma: a pilot study. J Nucl Med 2018;59(7):1076–80.

42. Heußer T, Mann P, Rank CM, et al. Investigation of the halo-artifact in 68Ga-PSMA-11-PET/MRI. PLoS One 2017;12(8):e0183329. Thierry B, ed.

43. Freitag MT, Kesch C, Cardinale J, et al. Simultaneous whole-body 18F–PSMA-1007-PET/MRI with integrated high-resolution multiparametric imaging of the prostatic fossa for comprehensive oncological staging of patients with prostate cancer: a pilot study. Eur J Nucl Med Mol Imaging 2018;45(3): 340–7.

44. Lee E, Park W, Ahn SH, et al. Interobserver variation in target volume for salvage radiotherapy in recurrent prostate cancer patients after radical prostatectomy using CT versus combined CT and MRI: a multicenter study (KROG 13-11). Radiat Oncol J 2018;36(1):11–6.

45. Villeirs GM, Van Vaerenbergh K, Vakaet L, et al. Interobserver delineation variation using CT versus combined CT + MRI in intensity–modulated radiotherapy for prostate cancer. Strahlenther Onkol 2005;181(7):424–30.

46. Kerkmeijer LGW, Maspero M, Meijer GJ, et al. Magnetic resonance imaging only workflow for radiotherapy simulation and planning in prostate cancer. Clin Oncol 2018;30(11):692–701.

47. Calais J, Czernin J, Cao M, et al. 68Ga-PSMA-11 PET/CT mapping of prostate cancer biochemical recurrence after radical prostatectomy in 270 patients with a PSA level of less than 1.0 ng/mL: impact on salvage radiotherapy planning. J Nucl Med 2018; 59(2):230–7.

48. Henkenberens C, Derlin T, Bengel FM, et al. Patterns of relapse as determined by 68Ga-PSMA ligand PET/CT after radical prostatectomy. Strahlenther Onkol 2018;194(4):303–10.

49. Habl G, Sauter K, Schiller K, et al. [68] Ga-PSMA-PET for radiation treatment planning in prostate cancer recurrences after surgery: individualized medicine or new standard in salvage treatment. Prostate 2017;77(8):920–7.

50. Stish BJ, Pisansky TM, Harmsen WS, et al. Improved metastasis-free and survival outcomes with early salvage radiotherapy in men with detectable prostate-specific antigen after prostatectomy for prostate cancer. J Clin Oncol 2016;34(32):3864–71.

51. Han S, Woo S, Kim YJ, et al. Impact of 68Ga-PSMA PET on the management of patients with prostate cancer: a systematic review and meta-analysis. Eur Urol 2018;74(2):179–90.

52. Grubmüller B, Baltzer P, D'Andrea D, et al. 68Ga-PSMA 11 ligand PET imaging in patients with biochemical recurrence after radical prostatectomy – diagnostic performance and impact on therapeutic decision-making. Eur J Nucl Med Mol Imaging 2018;45(2):235–42.

53. van Leeuwen PJ, Stricker P, Hruby G, et al. [68] Ga-PSMA has a high detection rate of prostate cancer recurrence outside the prostatic fossa in patients being considered for salvage radiation treatment. BJU Int 2016;117(5):732–9.

54. Bluemel C, Linke F, Herrmann K, et al. Impact of 68Ga-PSMA PET/CT on salvage radiotherapy planning in patients with prostate cancer and persisting PSA values or biochemical relapse after prostatectomy. EJNMMI Res 2016;6(1):78.

55. Zschaeck S, Wust P, Beck M, et al. Intermediate-term outcome after PSMA-PET guided high-dose radiotherapy of recurrent high-risk prostate cancer patients. Radiat Oncol 2017;12(1):140.

56. Sterzing F, Kratochwil C, Fiedler H, et al. 68Ga-PSMA-11 PET/CT: a new technique with high potential for the radiotherapeutic management of prostate cancer patients. Eur J Nucl Med Mol Imaging 2016;43(1):34–41.

57. Hope TA, Aggarwal R, Chee B, et al. Impact of 68Ga-PSMA-11 PET on management in patients with biochemically recurrent prostate cancer. J Nucl Med 2017;58(12):1956–61.

58. Afaq A, Alahmed S, Chen S-H, et al. Impact of 68Ga-prostate-specific membrane antigen PET/CT on prostate cancer management. J Nucl Med 2018;59(1):89–92.

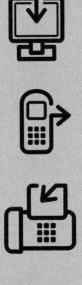

Printed and bound by CPI Group (UK) Ltd, Croydon, CR0 4YY

03/10/2024

01040308-0007